Residential Child Care Staff Selection: Choose with Care

Residential Child Care Staff Selection: Choose with Care has been co-published simultaneously as *Child & Youth Services*, Volume 23, Numbers 1/2 2001.

Residential Child Care Staff Selection: Choose with Care

Meredith Kiraly

Residential Child Care Staff Selection: Choose with Care has been co-published simultaneously as *Child & Youth Services*, Volume 23, Numbers 1/2 2001.

Routledge
Taylor & Francis Group
LONDON AND NEW YORK

Residential Child Care Staff Selection: Choose with Care has been co-published simultaneously as *Child & Youth Services*™, Volume 23, Numbers 1/2 2001.

First published 2001 by The Haworth Press, Inc.

This edition published 2016 by Routledge
2 Park Square, Milton Park, Abingdon, Oxon OX14 4RN
711 Third Avenue, New York, NY 10017, USA

Routledge is an imprint of the Taylor & Francis Group, an informa business

Library of Congress Cataloging-in-Publication Data

Kiraly, Meredith.
Residential child care staff selection: choose with care/Meredith Kiraly.
p. cm.
"Co-published simultaneously as Child & Youth Services, Volume 23, Numbers 1/2 2001."
Includes bibliographical references and index.
ISBN 0-7890-1745-8–ISBN 0-7890-1744-X
1. Child care workers–Selection and appointment. 2. Child care workers–Training of
3. Children–Institutional care. 4. Children–Institutional care–Israel. I. Title
HQ778.5 .K57 2002
362.71'2–dc21 2002014933

ISBN 13: 978-0-78901-745-1 (pbk)

Residential Child Care Staff Selection: Choose with Care

CONTENTS

ABOUT THE AUTHOR

Meredith Kiraly is a psychologist with twenty-five years experience in child and family programs in health, education, and welfare. In the last fifteen years she has been working in child, youth and family welfare services, particularly in residential care. She wrote this book while a program manager with MacKillop Family Services.

In the 1990s, she undertook a major research project on caregiver recruitment and selection. A Creswick Foundation Travelling Fellowship allowed her to visit the USA, the UK, Denmark, and Canada in 1994 to collect ideas from international authorities in both personnel selection and child/youth welfare. She has written *Recruiting and Selecting Residential Care Workers* (Kildonan Child and Family Services, 1999); *The Problem of the Paedophile: Guidelines for Recruiting Staff for Positions in Child and Youth Care,* a 1995 article for *Children Australia;* and other journal articles on youth welfare that have been published in Australia and the UK. She has also trained staff in recruitment and selection and given many conference papers on staff recruitment and other topics. She completed a Master of Behavioral Science on staff recruitment. She is currently doing project work for community services organizations, government, and tertiary institutions. Her e-mail address is <kiraly@melbpc.org.au>

SECTION A. STAFF SELECTION: A RESEARCH REPORT

Chapter 1

Introduction

> The best set of cottage parents I ever had was a pretty young couple . . . they were really understanding, both of them spent a lot of time with each kid, they really put in so much without being like, oh you know, "you poor little thing, I understand," sort of thing; they just had a lot of empathy for how you were feeling without actually having to go over the top like some of the social workers did, and they were a lot of fun. We always did a lot of fun things, and they tried to create a really normal atmosphere, which is really important, because when you go out and go to school you don't want everyone to know that your home is a bit strange compared to everybody else; it was very normal.
>
> *Young person in focus group*

This study explored the way staff are selected and supported to provide care to children and young people who, for whatever reason, find themselves living in residential care facilities for a period of their lives. It is part of an international movement to build excellence into residential child care and thus to improve options available for the care of children who have been the target of statutory intervention.

[Haworth co-indexing entry note]: "Introduction." Kiraly, Meredith. Co-published simultaneously in *Child & Youth Services* (The Haworth Press, Inc.) Vol. 23, No. 1/2, 2001, pp. 1-15; and: *Residential Child Care Staff Selection: Choose with Care* (Meredith Kiraly) The Haworth Press, Inc., 2001, pp. 1-15. Single or multiple copies of this article are available for a fee from The Haworth Document Delivery Service [1-800-HAWORTH 9:00 a.m. - 5:00 p.m. (EST). E-mail address: getinfo@haworthpressinc.com].

The push for quality in residential care is critical to the local context if vulnerable children and young people in our society are to be given the best chance for positive growth and development.

Specifically, the purpose of the project was to develop a model of best practice in residential child care staff selection. A preliminary step entailed identifying key factors that contribute to quality residential child care. In the course of the work some other issues emerged, and these were also explored, although in less detail. These include the importance of support measures needed for skilled staff to perform well and the question of training and professionalization of the residential child care industry.

Because this was a new and complex area of study with many variables, a naturalistic mode of inquiry was adopted with multiple methods of investigation. First, an extensive literature review focused on residential child care, personnel selection, and more broadly on child welfare. Then eight focus groups were conducted with four groups of stakeholders: young people who had been in care, parents of children who had been in care, residential child care workers, and supervisors of residential workers. A study tour was undertaken to North America, the United Kingdom, and Denmark in order to discuss relevant issues with authorities in personnel selection, residential child care, and related areas of child welfare.

Following these investigations, a pilot project explored the involvement of young people and parents in the staff selection process. These activities yielded a wealth of information that was analyzed for a profile of a skilled residential child care worker (see Appendix D) and a model of best practice in residential child care staff selection and support.

THE DEVELOPMENTAL NEEDS OF CHILDREN AWAY FROM HOME

Several authorities on substitute care have sought to identify the essential ingredients of good care for children for the out-of-home context. Fahlberg (1991), an authority on attachment and separation, says that the family provides:

- a primary caregiver for the child;
- care by specific adults to whom the child can become attached;
- continuous contact with these adults on a day-to-day basis;

- gradually changing relationships with a small number of individuals over a lifetime;
- safety and security;
- stimulation and encouragement for growth;
- reasonable expectations;
- experience in identifying and expressing emotions;
- support in times of stress; and
- others with whom to share successes. (p. 22)

Attachment is the medium through which the essential ingredients of care outlined above work to enable the satisfactory development of the growing child. Attachment has been defined as "an affectionate bond between two individuals that endures through space and time and serves to join them emotionally" (Fahlberg, 1991, p. 7). The carer's role is to help the child to develop healthy attachments so that continued growth and development are facilitated, and to aid in extending the attachments and behavioral gains achieved while in care to subsequent caregivers.

Maier (1979) identifies bodily comfort, differentiating between individuals, predictability, dependability, training in personal behavior, and care for the caregivers as the essential ingredients for the development of children away from home.

Beedell (Beedell & Clough, 1992) identified three main aspects of care: holding, nurturing, and the development and maintenance of personal integrity. *Holding* lies at the heart of the work. It implies solidity and security and includes processes to ensure survival and protection from danger and distress, and it involves elements of care, comfort, and control; it is the precondition for the rest of the activity in a home. *Nurturing* relates to all kinds of opportunities for growth, both formal and informal. It includes encouraging–and sometimes insisting on–the development of skills necessary for living. The *development of personal integrity* refers to the capacity of the person to become more fully integrated and to direct his or her life. It involves conveying societal norms about adult behavior, respect for an individual's own ways of meeting the demands of his or her life, and includes any restorative and therapeutic experience provided.

The role of the residential child care worker, then, entails striving to provide these conditions for a group of children who have been abused and/or neglected and who thus frequently display more than usually challenging behaviors. This is a challenging task indeed.

RESIDENTIAL CHILD CARE IN THE SPECTRUM OF SERVICES

Residential child care is one of a number of out-of-home care options. Like all forms of alternative care, it has its strengths and weaknesses. It is sometimes seen as more able to respond effectively to the needs of more challenging children than home-based care and/or as less likely to lead to placement breakdown. Further, some children and young people, if given a choice, will say that they prefer residential care to living with a family other than their own (Association of Child Welfare Agencies, 1992; Lindsay, personal communication, 1994). There are, nevertheless, disadvantages. It is, by and large, unable to provide permanent relationships and long-term commitment by caregivers to children, factors which are identified as critical to the healthy development of children (Goldstein, Freud, & Solnit, 1973). Placing together a group of abused and/or challenging children is often seen to be disadvantageous to their individual needs and development.

Recent child welfare policy developments in Australia, and especially in Victoria, favor a variety of foster care and other home-based care placements wherever possible, with a view to reducing the scope of residential child care to the smallest possible size (Department of Human Services, 1997; Health and Community Services, 1994). By contrast, in countries such as the United Kingdom and the United States, where the trend away from residential care occurred some years earlier than in Australia, there has been a move to reaffirm the role of residential care as a positive choice, to improve its status, and to give concerted attention to addressing the concerns which remain about its sometimes variable quality (Berridge, 1992a; Clough, 1994; Jamieson, 1994; Kahan, 1994; Magnuson, personal communication, 1994).

Whatever its place in the spectrum of services at any particular point in time, quality residential care is critical if children and young people in such placements are to be protected and develop well.

ABUSE IN CARE

Child welfare professionals and the community–via the media in recent years–are now aware that child abuse is a widespread issue in all forms of alternative care (Community Services Commission, 1996, p. 19). While local research in Australia on the incidence of abuse of children in out-of-home care is lacking (Cashmore, Dolby, & McGregor,

1994, p. 30), recent research in the United States has shown that the incidence of abuse of children by "stranger-caregivers," that is, in foster care, is reported at two to three times the rate of children living with their families (Nunno & Rindfleisch, 1991).

Concerns about the high rates of abuse in residential care have been long-standing in the United Kingdom (United Kingdom Department of Health, 1992, p. 20), where it is suggested that the problem tends to be widely denied or covered up (Cashmore, Dolby, & McGregor, 1994, p. 30).

The origins of abuse by care staff are many and complex. Some solutions may include an increase in funding levels, better training for staff, better accountability measures, changes in organizational climate and management, and improvements in staff support and management. In recent times, many local and overseas reports have drawn attention to the question of how to make the best assessments and decisions about selecting skilled staff. This area has become the focus of this study.

RESIDENTIAL CHILD CARE STAFF SELECTION

> Their hearts need to be in the right place.
>
> *Young person in focus group*

> Be careful about who you choose.
>
> *Young person in focus group*

Good staff are the backbone of residential child care. "As primary caregivers, residential child care workers have a key role to play in the quality of services for children in care" (Murphy, 1994, p. 27). An effective organization treats its workers as its most important asset (Peters & Waterman, 1986, p. 238). The skills and personal qualities of residential child care staff are the central features of quality care (Dill, 1990; Kahan, Banner, & Lane, 1986; Kahan & Levy, 1991; Skinner, 1994; Utting, 1991; Wagner, 1987). The best support and management, however, cannot result in good performance if the people employed do not have the required talent to perform the job. Talented staff can be trained and developed, but the talent itself cannot be created (Dill, 1990).

In an early publication on selecting staff for social care, Kahan, Banner, and Lane (1986) suggested that "Staff selection is always important, but never more so than when the personalities of the staff are part of their essential equipment needed to carry out the task" (p. 12). The process of coming to a staff selection decision is a complex one. In practice, the task is often undertaken with limited time and by people who are not specifically trained in the job. A popular myth is that it is all a matter of "gut feeling." Attention to the way these decisions are reached would thus appear to offer a critical opportunity to improve the quality of residential child care staffing.

In Australia, a number of local reports have directed attention to the subject of carer selection (Buzatu, 1987; Department of Community Welfare Services, 1985; Phillip Institute of Technology, 1982). However, no systematic research on the subject has been undertaken to date.

LINK TO HOME-BASED CARE RECRUITMENT

A range of home-based care programs now operate in Victoria. These include foster care, adolescent community placement, specialized home-based care, and lead tenant model care. These various programs provide community care for children and young people of different levels of challenge. While home-based care has many programmatic differences from residential care, an improved method of residential child care staff selection may have some aspects which are suitable for use in home-based carer selection.

PREVIOUS RESEARCH

There seems to be no other area of managerial practice where a large academic research literature has been as systematically ignored as it has been in the area of employee selection (Dreher & Maurer, 1989, p. 249).

The quest to find better methods of identifying quality staff has been the inspiration for nearly a century of research into personnel selection methods (Arvey and Campion, 1982). While much progress has been made, the integration of knowledge from research into personnel selection practices has been relatively slow. There are thus clear opportunities here for the residential child care field to improve its staff selection practices.

A substantial amount of research information specifically on the topic of residential child care staff selection has also been published in the United States in the last 20 years. This body of information consists mainly of a series of small and unrelated research projects in which a variety of psychometric tests have been used as selection instruments in addition to the traditional employment interview. However, none of this research has been translated into a consistent code of practice for residential child care staff selection.

In the United Kingdom, a major push toward the development of standards in residential child care staff selection and management appeared after the commencement of this research project in 1990. It emanated from scandals in recent years about poor practices in residential care that culminated in a series of inquiries (United Kingdom Department of Health, 1992). One of the most serious of these scandals, which led to a review of staff selection and management practices, was directly related to the activities of a pedophile, Frank Beck. Beck was employed as the head of a children's home and was subsequently convicted of numerous sexual and other offences against children in the home. After coming to the attention of authorities because of malpractice in one post, he was able to again obtain employment in another position in the residential child care field. This incident led to the Warner Inquiry into staff selection and management in children's homes and to the establishment of the *Support Force for Children's Residential Care* (1994; 1995a; 1995b), which produced a series of publications on related topics. The Support Force also focused upon linking United Kingdom Local Authorities with each other in order to share practice developments in residential care.

THE PROBLEM OF THE PEDOPHILE

Much of the recent energy surrounding the interest in staff selection in the United Kingdom was thus focused on detecting and deterring child abusers. As a result of this, child welfare authorities in the United Kingdom and Canada have warned of international pedophile rings that are likely to become evident in residential child care in this country and others (Kahan, personal communication, 1994; Lindsay, personal communication, 1994; Meston, personal communication, 1994). Thus, while the initiative for this project in 1990 was not related to these concerns, it is now clear that the risk of recruiting abusive staff needs to be addressed.

STAFF SUPPORT

While staff selection is critical to the provision of good care, it cannot alone guarantee this. In the United Kingdom and the United States, there is some concern that the current focus on staff selection practices presumes that good selection practice can eliminate most staffing problems (Clough, 1994; Platt, personal communication, 1994; Stuck, personal communication, 1994). These authorities have expressed concern that attention to staff selection practices in residential child care has the potential to divert attention away from other areas of staff support and management. Thus, while the main focus of this project is staff selection, some attention has also been given to the question of staff support in the course of the investigation.

ORIGINS OF THE STUDY

The research that forms the substance of this thesis has arisen out of my twelve years of practice in the residential child care field. The residential care program of Kildonan Homes for Children (later Kildonan Child and Family Services), a Uniting Church agency in the inner city of Melbourne, provided the opportunity for this work. Over a number of years, the program had been progressively reviewed and developed with a focus on improving the quality of care offered.

It was in this context that staff selection presented itself as an issue that seemed to warrant more careful attention. The management team became aware that they had little theoretical knowledge relating to personnel selection and no clear basis for deciding what the qualities of a skilled residential child care worker might be. On occasion it seemed that less than ideal care might have had its origins in a hurried or uncertain selection process.

The focus of attention in this research project thus became how to select the best carers with the aim of improving quality of care. This contrasts then to some extent with the focus of the British work in staff selection that paralleled this work from 1992 to 1995, whose goals were preventing abuse.

The outcome of this research has been to develop a working model of residential child care staff selection and support, recognizing that a good selection process cannot stand alone without ongoing and effective staff support processes.

FIELD HANDBOOKS BASED ON THIS WORK

This research project has also led to the writing of two handbooks for staff working in the direct care of children and young people. The first is *Recruiting and Selecting Residential Care Workers* (Kildonan Child and Family Services, 1999). This handbook provides an accessible guide to the model of residential child care staff selection and support developed through this project. The second is *Choose with Care: A Recruitment Guide for Organizations Working with Children*, originally published by ECPAT (End Child Prostitution, Pornography and Trafficking) Australia and MacKillop Family Services in 1999. This latter handbook is included in this volume as the concluding document.

CONTEXT

A number of contextual issues impact upon a consideration of questions regarding residential child care staff selection. Some of these issues are described below, setting the scene for the literature review and subsequent development of the research questions.

The Image of Residential Child Care

The greatest barrier to establishing good standards in the recruitment and selection of residential child care staff is the poor status of residential child care in Australia and across the English-speaking world.

> Respondents to our survey from all sectors report recruitment difficulties arising from the unattractive image of residential child care. Employers say that the main contributing factors to this unattractive image are poor pay, limited training and career development opportunities, insufficient recognition of and compensation for anti-social hours, inadequate supervision, and unsatisfactory support arrangements. The point was starkly put by one employer that recruitment problems arose from "the association of residential child care with poorly paid women's work." (United Kingdom Department of Health, 1992, p. 25)

The system is little different in Australia. In a study of the needs of residential child care workers in Melbourne, Murphy (1994) states:

> It is a common perception that residential care is the last and least desirable option–to be used only when all other approaches to provide care and protection for children have been tried first. The field's current practice of staffing residential facilities with inexperienced, untrained and undertrained personnel, providing them with an inadequate salary and virtually no career structure, suggests that agencies consider that little can be done for those children who finally reach the "last alternative" and who, therefore, only warrant a minimum allocation of resources to provide for their care. . . (p. 32)

Attention to staff selection practices needs to be seen in the context of the low status of residential child care in the Australian child welfare field. Real improvement in this area can only take place in the context of improving standards in residential child care and its image in general. As Kahan (1994) says, "Poor staff selection is all of a piece with the Cinderella role of residential care."

Current Threats from Fiscally-Driven Child Protection Policy

Like other local and national governments, Victoria is currently in the throes of substantial cutbacks to funding for child welfare and, in particular, residential child care, in part because of its high cost. In Australia, home-based care (foster care and its variants) is now seen as the placement of choice, and residential care as the placement of last resort. Threats to quality residential care from this funding climate may include limited staffing models and staff support and restrictions on the availability of an appropriate range of residential placement options.

The drive to more economical forms of response to children at risk has, however, led to some creative programmatic initiatives that are good practice and cost-effective alternatives. In addition to innovations in home-based care, significant developments have been made in establishing a range of models of Intensive Home-Based Services (IFBS). Family Group Conferencing, originating in New Zealand and developed further in Australia, has provided another powerful alternative way to respond to allegations of abuse. These new programmatic options work best, however, when driven by case-specific needs and when a range of care options remain for those children and young people who still need them.

Moves the Direction of Family-Centered Practice

A recent shift in child welfare practice has been towards the greater recognition of the importance of continuing relationships with the birth family for the development and well-being of children in care. Practice that supports family contact with separated children and to improving the living circumstances and functioning of families provides significantly improved opportunities for family reunification for children in care and/or family connection and support in adult life. This view is encapsulated in the assumption "[That] child and family are irrevocably linked and that the best long term interests of the child can only be guaranteed by ensuring that birth parent(s) and family members continue to be respected and have a place in their child(ren)'s daily life" (Ainsworth & Small, 1994, p. 23).

The day-to-day practice of residential care and its management can go a long way towards effecting family support and reconnection. Contact between family members and children in care needs to be facilitated; interventions should recognize the importance of family to children, and agency policy and procedures should include processes to include family members and their input.

Family-centered practice has many implications for the staffing of residential child care units. Staff must be positively-oriented towards the families of children in care. They need to be non-judgmental with good communication skills, appropriate training in working with family as part of the child care task, the support of a supervising case worker in guiding and sharing the associated tasks, and they must be able to manage these new job requirements within the time and resources available. This is discussed further below.

The Changing Nature of the Job

Research into personnel selection emphasizes repeatedly the need to be clear about what the job entails (Equal Employment Opportunity Commission, 1978; Lathan, Saari, Pursell, & Campion, 1980; Pecora & Austin, 1987; Pfau, 1990). A key question is thus the changing expectations of residential child care workers in today's service system. Twenty years ago, a residential child care worker was charged with the direct care of larger numbers of children than today. However, the direct care of these children was more or less the whole job. Today, many more tasks–calling on a variety of skills–are being expected of the worker. New requirements include working more inclusively with the families of children in care (as described above), managing household budgets, writing reports, and policy and program development. More responsibility, autonomy, and professionalism are being accorded to the residential worker. With the recent closure of many residential units, those children and young people remaining in care tend to have more challenging behaviors that staff are expected to manage effectively and within the guidelines of acceptable child care practices.

The ever-increasing demands and sophistication of the job of residential child care worker suggest that the industry needs to pay much more attention to training staff than in the past. The development of specific training courses for residential workers in some countries has been a major step forward for the residential child care field. However, hopes that such courses would provide minimum standards for residential child care employment have not yet been realized, and funding constraints threaten progress towards a trained residential child care work-force via both pre-service and in-service training. Nevertheless, child welfare practitioners are increasingly seeing comprehensive training–both pre-service and in-service–as essential to the ever-increasing complexities of residential child care work.

Models of Care: Rostered Units and Family Group Homes

The performance quality of care staff is the model of care in which they will work. Rostered staffing models offer better working conditions and stress relief for staff than do family group homes. Continuity and consistency of care are, however, harder to achieve than in a family group home. A key issue for rostered units is the capacity to generate and maintain a cooperative team approach to service delivery in order to maximize the quality and consistency of care. The impact of different models of care on staff and residents needs to be considered in the quest to improve care. The skills needed to perform well in the role of residential care worker in a family group home may differ somewhat from those needed to perform as a rostered residential care worker; selection processes will need to reflect these differences. For example, a rostered worker may need to have stronger teamwork skills than a family group home carer; conversely, a family group home carer may need greater endurance and resilience to cope with the long shifts and solo work. Also, supports to staff need to vary according to the model.

The Family Group Home Model

This model of care is still very prevalent in Victoria and some other Australian states. A family group home is usually run by a couple working together to provide care to a small group of children. In most cases only one member of the couple is formally employed and the other operates as a part-time volunteer, or they are paid together as part of a compensation and benefit package. A common feature of the model is that the birth children of the staff may live in the family group home. This model is largely superseded in the United Kingdom (Berridge & Brophy, personal communication, 1994) and the United States (Magnuson, personal communication, 1994). However, in Victoria it has developed, over time, to become the vehicle for care of some of the most challenging children and young people in the protective system.

Changes in the model have been wrought by a changing society and the difficulties of recruiting suitable staff. Increasingly, agencies are employing single people and staff with immediate family living in who do not conform to the conventional nuclear family model (e.g., unmarried couples, couples with a step-child). Staffing levels in family group homes have, however, increased little since the 1950s. The family group home is likely to remain a common model of care in the foreseeable future, at least in part because it is much cheaper to fund than alternative forms of residential care. It will, however, need substantial additional resourcing if it is to provide good quality care for increasingly challenging placements.

Despite resourcing problems, the family group home offers a level of consistency and continuity of care unmatched in other forms of residential care, assuming that staff burnout and turnover can be controlled. However, a number of other concerns have also been raised in regard to the model. The long continuous shifts (e.g., 24 hours per day of responsibility or working from 5-26 days straight) may generate ongoing stress and a loss of objectivity for staff, in addition to burnout. Problems sometimes arise around the role of the "volunteer" spouse, such as a lack of accountability and claims of exploitation of volunteer labor. Marital difficulties may be generated by the work, with significant stress for the employee and all in the unit.

There are also a series of issues relating to the presence of the staff's children in the residential unit. The child-to-staff ratio under this model, officially set at around 4 to 1, may rise substantially when the children of the family group home carer are included. Multiple life tasks (marriage, child-raising, and child care work) are played out in the work domain. While field experience sometimes bears witness to benefits in this family-like arrangement, it also has the capacity to generate a number of problems. Incompatibility of the needs and behaviors of resident children and staff's children may lead to conflicts of personal and professional interests for staff. Carers need to be able simultaneously to look after the needs of their own dependent children, those of the children in care, and themselves, under very challenging conditions. This is a "big ask." When care falls below acceptable levels, issues relating to the compatibility of the carer's family life issues with the demands of the job may become confused with the question of the suitability of the carer for the position.

The family group home thus presents complex issues for staff selection. First, the partner needs to be selected for his or her unusual volunteer status. Second, agencies normally attempt to make some assessment of the strength and effectiveness of the marital relationship and teamwork, a particularly optimistic goal for the selection interview. The children of staff living-in pose, however, possibly the most complex problem for recruitment and selection in terms of assessing their suitability for family group home life; yet much of the carers' capacity to perform well may depend on the individual needs of each of their own children and whether these can be met "on the job."

Because of the complexity of this issue and its potential to affect the performance of the carer, the question of birth children of staff living in the family group home is addressed separately.

Children's Rights

One of the characteristics of organizational excellence is said to be the capacity of an organization to stay close to the consumer. This attribute is defined as "the process of learning from people you serve by listening intently and regularly" (Pecora & Austin, 1987, p. 11). Characteristically, such an organization will involve consumers in all aspects of innovation and growth (Janz, Hellervik, & Gilmore, 1986, p. 45).

Children's rights have been receiving considerable attention in the child welfare field in Australia, Canada, and the United Kingdom in recent years and are now reflected in legislation in both Australia and the United Kingdom (United Kingdom, 1989; Victoria, 1989). The recent development of local consumer groups such as the Australian Association of Young People in Care (AAYPIC) and its state counterparts, based upon British and Canadian models, are other ways in which children and young people in residential care are being empowered. Children and young people need to be assisted to speak out on their own behalf and to have their issues addressed appropriately (A. B. & Y. Z., personal communication, 1994; AAYPIC, 1994; Lindsay, 1995). Feedback from consumers needs to be actively solicited in a variety of ways about their needs and wishes, allowing for better information on which to plan both day-to-day care and program developments. A recognition of children's rights predicates the need to create processes that will facilitate children and young people being more able to make complaints about abuse by care staff (A. B. & Y. Z., personal communication, 1994; Lindsay, personal communication, 1994; Platt, personal communication, 1994; Willow, 1996).

Developments in the implementation of the rights of children in care have influenced the methodology of this program and led to further exploration of this issue in relation to residential care staffing. A specific application is to explore the involvement of young people in staff selection (see Kiraly, 1998).

Chapter 2

Background

A premise of this work was that literature from the human resources management field, in particular the literature on personnel selection, would inform the question of how to best select residential child care staff. A major focus was literature on the employment interview, which was at this stage understood to be the central focus of the selection process. An exploration of published material specifically on residential child care staff selection followed from this. A further focus was literature that might inform the choice of an appropriate research methodology.

PERSONNEL SELECTION METHODS

There is a vast body of research literature on the subject of personnel selection; much of it focuses on the employment interview, but it also includes job analysis, psychological testing, the reference check, and other employment assessment methods.

Job Analysis

The process of selecting a worker to perform a particular job requires that management is clear about the nature of the job and the specific skills or characteristics required by the worker.

The objective of the job analysis is to generate a description of the job in terms of required knowledge, skills, abilities, and other worker characteristics. The job analysis should lead to both a clear job description and person specification (McLaughlin & McLean, 1987). In the United States, this process is legally required to ensure that jobs are clearly de-

---

[Haworth co-indexing entry note]: "Background." Kiraly, Meredith. Co-published simultaneously in *Child & Youth Services* (The Haworth Press, Inc.) Vol. 23, No. 1/2, 2001, pp. 17-49; and: *Residential Child Care Staff Selection: Choose with Care* (Meredith Kiraly) The Haworth Press, Inc., 2001, pp. 17-49. Single or multiple copies of this article are available for a fee from The Haworth Document Delivery Service [1-800-HAWORTH 9:00 a.m. - 5:00 p.m. (EST). E-mail address: getinfo@haworthpressinc.com].

fined and that the employer can demonstrate that selection methods are actually related to performance of the job in question (see Dessler, 1988, p. 77; Equal Employment Opportunity Coordinating Council, 1976, p. 51738). Pursell, Campion, and Gaylord (1980) state that there is evidence that selection systems based on job analysis are more valid and less biased against minority groups. This finding is echoed by Wiesner and Cronshaw (1988), who found that studies using a formal job analysis produced higher validities than did studies using an informal job analysis.

Pursell, Campion, and Gaylord (1980) comment that while various techniques may be used to collect information, job analysis participants should be selected on the basis of their extensive knowledge of the job and should include both supervisors and incumbents. Specific job-duty and job-requirement information should be produced; the job should be described as it currently is, not how it might be changed or improved, and all job requirements needed to perform all the specific job duties should be specified. Job duties can then be ranked on their importance to job success and in terms of the amount of time they take. The knowledge, skills; attitudes, and other characteristics are then identified for each of the job duties.

Pfau (1990) cites inaccurate job analysis as one of the ten most common interviewing mistakes. Researchers on the *Situational Interview* (Latham, Saari, Pursell, & Campion, 1980) stress that a systematic job analysis is used to develop this interview *pro forma*, as well as their performance appraisal.

Possibly conflicting with Pursell, Campion, and Gaylord (1980), Schneider and Konz (1989) advocate a strategic or future-oriented approach in order to take into account both present and future needs. This would appear to be particularly relevant to the residential child care field at the present time.

Pecora and Austin (1987) stress the importance of the process of job analysis to develop job descriptions in human services and provide a detailed description of how to go about this. They recommend the use of specific, detailed, and behaviorally-defined task statements to make up job descriptions, and they supply examples of a "task bank" to assist with these. While a complex and time consuming task, it is defended as an important basis for the recruitment and selection process.

Residential child care workers' jobs vary greatly from one place to another. Job analysis is thus a crucial consideration for the selection of care staff.

The Employment Interview

Wiesner and Cronshaw (1988) define the employment interview as:

> . . . an interpersonal interaction of limited duration between one or more interviewers and a job-seeker for the purpose of identifying interviewee knowledge, skills, abilities and behaviors that may be predictive of success in subsequent employment. The operational indicators of this success include criteria of job performance, training success, promotion and tenure. (p. 276)

The use of the employment interview as the primary method of staff selection persists across all industries, despite a now overwhelming body of literature that has shown, repeatedly, that the validity of the traditional employment interview is extremely low. For example, Arvey and Campion (1982) describe the problems of individual interviewer bias and a lack of clear job analysis as possible causes of problems, and they recommend panel interviewing and more attention to job analysis as solutions. Other writers have focused on the lack of structure in interviewing as a more critical factor in generating poor validity (Pursell, Campion, & Gaylord, 1980; Wiesner & Cronshaw, 1988). With such evidence of validity problems, the employment interview merits close examination if better selection practice is to be effected.

Historical context

The employment interview has been studied as far back as 1915. Prior to the second World War, little research into its reliability and validity was undertaken. During the war years, large groupings of military recruits provided both the need and the opportunity for work on the validation of selection procedures for military service of various kinds, such as pilots and naval electricians (Eder, Kacmar, & Ferris, 1989). However, probably the single most significant impetus for personnel selection research has been the passage of the *United States Civil Rights Act* (Giffin, 1989; United States of America, 1964). Research into whether tests and interview procedures that were developed for a predominantly white, male workforce could be used for women and minorities began in earnest following this landmark event. The Equal Employment Opportunity Act (United States of America, 1972) led to vigorous enforcement of Title VII of the Civil Rights Act and directed researchers' attention to the interview's legal liability. Issues of fairness were added to issues of reliability and validity, and research on gender bias became particularly plentiful (Eder, Kacmar, & Ferris, 1989, p. 26). Litigation arising from Title VII led to increased employer concern with selection procedures.

A further legal development significantly affecting research into selection methods was the *Uniform Guidelines on Employee Selection Procedures* (Equal Employment Opportunity Commission, 1978). These guidelines define stringent procedural and documentation requirements for the design and implementation of personnel selection systems (Pursell, Campion, & Gaylord, 1980). These events in the U.S. explain why most of the research studies originate there.

Numerous aspects of the employment interview have been studied over the last twenty years. The results of these investigations were reported in a number of reviews. The most recent and significant are articles by Arvey and Campion (1982), Weisner and Cronshaw (1988), and Harris (1989). These articles have reviewed literature covering a range of issues in employment interviewing. Some of the major areas reviewed include reliability and validity of the employment interview, applicant characteristics (including questions of bias against minority groups and gender bias), interviewer decision-making, methodological issues, and interviewer training.

Improvements in reliability and validity: The structured interview

The research on the reliability and validity of the employment interview is the most significant and meaningful. Until recently, a large body of research has suggested that the employment interview is not a valid indicator of job performance (Arvey & Campion, 1982; Campion, Pursell, & Brown, 1988; Zedeck, Tziner, & Middlestadt, 1983).

In recent years, however, significant advances appear to have been made in relation to improving validity. These advances point consistently to the crucial importance of structuring the employment interview to ensure job relevance and consistency of application.

The structured interviewing process has the following characteristics:

- It is based exclusively on job duties and requirements that are critical to job performance.
- It has four different types of questions which may be used: situational questions, job knowledge questions, job sample/simulation questions, and worker requirement questions.

- It is actually a selection test and may include three sections: oral, written and physical.
- It has sample answers to each question determined in advance. Interviewee responses are rated on a 5-point scale defined explicitly in advance.
- It has an interview committee so that the interviewee responses are evaluated by multiple raters. . .
- It is consistently applied to each applicant. For example, the same committee members are used; one member asks all the questions each time; and the same scoring method is used.
- It is documented for future reference and in case of legal challenge . . . (Campion, Pursell, and Brown, 1988, p. 908)

Weisner and Cronshaw's (1988) meta-analysis of 150 other studies found that the structured interview had on average a corrected validity coefficient of 0.62, a quite respectable validity for a selection method.

One of the earlier attempts at consistent structuring of the interview was the Situational Interview (SI), devised in 1980, with its authors claiming significant advances in reliability and validity (Latham, Saari, Pursell, & Campion, 1980; Latham & Saari, 1984; Pursell, Campion, & Gaylord, 1980). The SI has structured questions about how an applicant would respond to various situations. It is suggested that a carefully-designed situational interview, in which the answers to questions are not obvious, can produce higher validity coefficients (0.30-0.50) than any other interview methods, and begin to compare with the validity coefficients from cognitive ability testing.

By 1988, a series of studies identified the improved validity of the structured interview over the unstructured interview (Maurer & Fay, 1988; Wiesner & Cronshaw, 1988; Wright, Lichtenfels & Pursell, 1989). Wiesner and Cronshaw (1988) made a series of recommendations for future research:

1. Researchers should divert their attention from the unstructured to the structured interview. . .
2. Researchers should concentrate on identifying factors moderating the validity of the structured interview with the goal of maximizing the validity of the structured interview. Two promising factors identified in *post hoc* analyses are improvement of interview reliability and the use of formal job-analytic information for developing structured questions.

3. Industrial/organizational psychologists should discard the "received doctrine" of interview invalidity. . . .
4. Practitioners should use the structured interview (as opposed to the unstructured interview) wherever possible. The structured interview questions should be based on formal job-analytic information and every attempt should be made to maximize the reliability of the structured interview.
5. When using structured board interviews, the consensus board may be preferable to the statistical combination of individual board member ratings. Further research should be conducted to understand *why* consensus boards seem to yield superior prediction. (p. 289)

Weisner and Cronshaw's comments about the consensus board are, however, contradicted by other research in the field (Anderson, personal communication, 1994; Fletcher, 1994). These researchers strongly advocate making decisions based upon arithmetic ratings undertaken by individual panel members prior to any discussion and group decision-making process.

A variant on the structured interview is the *Patterned Behavioral Description Interview* (PBDI) (Janz, 1982). The PBDI relies on questions asking how the applicant has responded in the past to these situations. Janz claimed a validity coefficient of 0.54 for this method, although he acknowledged some methodological flaws in this research. It would seem that it may not be a fully structured interview, in that different questions may be asked of different applicants. The PBDI gained some popularity in the 1980s and has been used in training programs (for example, Melrose Film Productions, 1994). Some controversy exists in the literature as to whether the SI or the PBDI is more valid.

The effect of applicant characteristics on selection outcomes

As already mentioned, discrimination and Equal Employment Opportunity (EEO) issues led to much of the research on the employment interview, including study of bias. Arvey (1979) noted that gender bias was particularly significant in most of the studies, compared to race, handicap, and age.

The evidence regarding other forms of discrimination then was less plentiful and less clear. However, by 1989 the evidence of gender bias also seemed less clear. Harris' meta-analysis of the employment interview (1989) reveals that more recent studies have not yielded clear evidence of gender discrimination in selection interviewing. Harris commented that it is not clear whether discrimination against women was in fact less prevalent in general or whether these research studies used settings and stimuli that provided a great deal of job-related qualifications information, thus minimizing the incidence of discrimination.

Campion and Arvey (1989) reported evidence of bias against men in the employment interview when the job is regarded as stereotypically female, and some evidence that women were discriminated against more when fewer applied for a given position. Similar findings were noted for older job applicants.

The question of racial discrimination has also been studied over this period; however, results have been conflicting, and at the present time, more work is needed on this issue before a general picture comes clear. The same applies to work on age and disability discrimination (Harris, 1989).

Other studies have addressed a large range of applicant characteristics such as non-verbal behavior in interviews (Rasmussen, 1984), applicants' dress (Forsythe, Drake, & Cox, 1985), and impression management (Gilmore & Ferris, 1989).

Interviewer training

A continuing research concern about the Situational Interview was the problem of interviewer inter-rater reliability, which affects and limits the validity of the interview process. Interviewers frequently vary in the way they rate interview performance. Some consistently rate high or low. Halo and Horns effects–that is, giving unduly high or low overall ratings because of one salient feature, for example, charm, untidy dress, appear to be common. Training would seem to be the answer to these problems; however, interviewer training is another difficult and confusing area, with conflicting results (Harris, 1989).

Earlier studies of this topic (Latham, Wexley, & Pursell, 1975; Wexley, Sanders, & Yukl, 1973) bear witness to the difficulty of establishing clearly the benefits of training interviewers to avoid rater errors such as halo, central tendency, and leniency. The only successful methods of training demonstrated in these two studies were the use of videotaped interview performances which were then ranked by the trainees, with results being discussed and the "correct" ratings given. The studies suggested that training may be better oriented towards establishing expected standards, accurate observation, and adequate definition of performance standards rather than towards rater error per se. Indeed, apparent rater effects such as leniency may, under some circumstances, reflect more accurate observations than normally scattered scores, due to the nature of the populations being evaluated, such as candidates short-listed for interviewing who may have been already selected as largely better than average (Bernardin & Pence, 1980). More recently, Maurer and Fay (1988) found no significant training effect despite the use of an 8-hour workshop format. This was, however, a study with a small sample size.

Arvey and Campion (1982) commented that while most research had focused on rater accuracy training, possibly other dimensions of interviewer behavior should become the subject of training, such as interpersonal skills and questioning styles. In reviewing recent literature, Harris (1989) noted that little has been published in this area in recent years and suggested that there is a need for a study directly comparing different interview training methods and using various criteria of effectiveness.

Interviewer decision-making

A number of researchers have studied how interviewers come to decisions about selecting employees. Arvey and Campion (1982) concluded that there was still evidence from studies conducted in the 1970s that interviewers tend to produce ratings that are influenced by contrast, primacy-recency, first impressions, personal feelings, and other factors. On the positive side, some research indicates that when evaluations are in the form of specific predictions of job behavior, less distortion is found.

One area of particular relevance to practice is research on the effect of previewing the application form on interview process and outcomes. Dipboye, Fontenelle, and Garner (1984) found that giving information on candidates via previewing the application form biased both the conduct of the interview and the processing of information-gathering in the interview. They concluded that if the interviewer is making judgments of the interviewee's qualifications for the job, it is better to avoid previewing the application form. On the other hand, if the primary function is to gather additional information, it is appropriate to preview the application. Regarding methodology, it is worth noting that the interviews were simulated, and that ratings were made by observers, not interviewers, and that the interviews had a low degree of structure. Tucker and Rowe (1979) found that previewing an unfavorable letter of reference biased judgments about interview data.

Dipboye (1989) claims that it is a fact that post-interview impressions tend to conform to pre-interview impressions, and that "the interview seems most likely to contribute to the prediction of a criterion to the extent that the information gathered during this phase is kept independent of information gathered in the first phase and considered on its own merit" (p. 49). Moreover, "It is abundantly clear that whatever information occurs first has a disproportionate influence on the final outcome of interviews" (Hakel, cited in Dipboye, 1989, p. 52).

In two studies of confirmatory bias, where subjects (i.e., interviewers) were allowed to generate their own questions, confirmatory bias was found. Binning, Goldstein, Garcia, Harding, and Scattaregia (1988) report that applicants who appeared poorly qualified were asked fewer questions about positive points than more highly qualified candidates. In addition, less qualified candidates were asked more difficult questions than qualified candidates. Macan and Dipboye (1988) reported that the results were more complex: Subjects were more likely to ask positive questions of highly qualified candidates of the same sex, but they were also more likely to ask positive questions of less qualified candidates of the opposite sex. Binning et al. (1988) suggest that such results are another strong argument for structuring the interview format as recommended by writers such as Latham, Saari, Pursell, and Campion (1980) and Wiesner and Cronshaw (1988). However, Binning, Goldstein, Garcia, Harding, and Scattaregia (1988) point out that "even the most structured interview systems do not eliminate or fully control the role of follow-up questioning as a valuable information-gathering strategy. Departures from a structured format, in the form of follow-up questioning, could be susceptible to confirmatory effects as well" (p. 35).

Another area of decision-making is the length of time interviewers take to make a decision. A popular management myth that has been perpetuated since a study in the 1950s (Springbett, 1958) is that interviewers typically make "snap" decisions within the first few minutes of the interview. This has been shown in several subsequent studies not to be the case (Buckley & Eder, 1988); however, the time taken to make a decision seems to vary according to a complex set of variables. In one of these subsequent studies, Tullar, Mullins, and Caldwell (1979) found that the interviewers took significantly longer to make a decision when interviewing a high-quality applicant. They also took more time to decide when they expected the interview to last longer by comparison with shorter interviewers. Tullar, Mullins, and Caldwell suggested that the longer a decision is delayed, the more likely it will be based on complete information. Allotting more time for a given interview may make the interviewer less likely to make a premature decision.

In a study of police officer selection, Furnham and Burnbeck (1989) concluded that the greater the interviewer's job experience (in years) or interviewing experience, the stricter (less generous) were his/her ratings.

The employment interview as a communication device

All of the above research is predicated upon a view of the selection interview as a one-way information-gathering technique in which the interviewer is responsible for eliciting enough accurate information from the applicant on which to make a valid selection decision. This view is known as the "objectivist-psychometric perspective." An alternative view stresses the interactional nature of the interview where the applicant and interviewer are actively negotiating for a desired outcome and that each is making decisions about their future. This view is known as the "subjectivist-social perception perspective." In this view, the interview is seen as effective not merely to the extent that the interviewer's ratings predict successful job performance but to the extent to which it facilitates the negotiation of the psychological contract between employer and employee (Anderson, 1992).

The "subjectivist-social perception perspective" explains the continued popularity of the selection interview despite concerns with its objective reliability and validity, because it is in fact serving a more crucial social purpose. For this reason, it will remain in almost universal usage and deserves attention in order to reduce the potential sources of error.

> Managers resist abandoning unstructured interviews because they are convinced that this class of techniques provides useful information about job candidates and helps achieve other important organizational objectives. These objectives and perceptions should play a more integral part in future employment interview research. (Dreher & Maurer, 1989, p. 268)

Anderson (1992) says that areas for future research that reflect this view include impression management by both interviewers and interviewees, the treatment of disfunction in interviewer information processing and decision-making, and the effects of different distributions of situational power upon interview processes and outcomes.

Psychological Testing

The lack of confidence of researchers in the validity of the employment interview led to a search for other, more apparently "scientific" and, hopefully, more statistically valid ways of selecting staff. A major alternative is psychological testing. This push has been linked to a growing industry of specialized psychological testing services, keen to promote their products (Fletcher, 1993).

Beach (cited in Pecora, 1987, p. 41) offers a series of guidelines regarding the use of tests as employee selection devices. These include using tests as a supplement to rather than a replacement for other selection devices, using tests to pick a select group from a much larger group, validating tests in one's own organization, using tests where it is difficult to obtain satisfactory employees through other selection methods, not viewing tests as precise and exact measures of the characteristic being tested, and not viewing high test scores as necessarily better predictors of satisfactory job performance than slightly lower scores.

Research into psychological testing falls into two main areas: intelligence (or cognitive) testing and personality testing.

Intelligence testing and personnel selection

Cognitive aptitude (general intelligence) has been proven to be the best predictor of job performance yet known (Barrett & Depinet, 1991; Hunter, 1986). However, Arvey (1986) and Gottfredson (1986) suggest that jobs themselves may require different levels of general cognitive functioning and cognitive aptitude testing may be more or less valid in predicting performance depending upon the job itself.

A contrary view of testing for personnel selection has persisted in both popular writing and professional psychology texts since the 1970s. This view was based on the work of McClelland (1973) who asserted that educational attainment and intelligence test scores did not predict occupational success, were unfair to minorities, and should be discarded in favor of specific testing of "competencies." Arvey (1986) questions whether several research methods may have contributed to the apparently poor results in the research on competency testing. He suggests that more specific criterion measures against which competencies may be validated and the use of larger samples in research studies may generate more respectable validities. With issues of fairness remaining prominent in both current debate and legislation, more work is needed in this area.

While a controversial area, what seems clear is that global intelligence may be a more important factor in work performance in general than is often recognized.

Personality testing

Personality tests have had a place in personnel selection for many years, in particular in the business world and in executive selection. The question of personality testing in staff selection is particularly pertinent to residential child care staff selection. Numerous small studies have attempted to solve the problem of how to select the best residential care staff by this means.

Current research literature suggests that personality tests may, under the best circumstances of appropriate use and skilled administration, offer modest incremental validity to the personnel selection process (Barrick &

Mount, 1991; Robertson & Makin, 1993), up to about .26 (Fletcher, 1991), substantially lower than that for cognitive ability tests. However, like the employment interview and other selection devices, application of personality testing frequently falls short of adequate standards, and it is partly because of this that much skepticism surrounds their use.

A vehement case against the use of personality testing in personnel selection was made by Stone (1985). Stone pointed out that personality tests were not designed for personnel work but for clinical diagnosis, that they are frequently normed on different populations than those typical of employment applicants, that they are difficult to validate as personnel selection tools, that they are subject to "faking," and are discriminatory. In a more recent publication, edited by Fletcher (1991), personnel practitioners Steve Blinkhorn and Charles Johnson (1991) argued that personality tests have insufficient validity compared to ability and aptitude testing. Six British experts in the field of personnel selection opposed this position. Robertson cited two meta-analyses demonstrating an acceptable, if limited, level of validity for the use of personality tests and claimed that even limited validity for this method, in conjunction with other selection methods, can be useful in improving the hit rate in selection.

Smith outlined three reasons why the issue is clouded. The first is the inclusion of some "wacky" personality measures, such as inkblot tests; the second is the problem of criteria also being of limited validity (for example, supervisors' ratings), and the third is that data is rarely available for all who complete the test, since only the best are selected. He also suggested that combining test scales may be more useful than single scales and stressed the importance of a trained and experienced test user.

The other question in relation to personality testing relates to which psychological characteristics are sought and tested for. Barrick and Mount (1991) suggest using a constellation of five major personality factors which are relatively robust and which have been explored in terms of their contribution to job performance. These five factors are extraversion, emotional stability, agreeableness, conscientiousness and openness to experience. Of these, the one that is linked clearly to a number of job performance criteria in all occupational groups is *conscientiousness. Emotional stability* proved to have little correlation with job performance and in professional groups actually appeared to have a negative correlation with performance. In context, it may be that the selected persons had sufficient emotional stability to do the job and that, beyond a certain range, "more was not necessarily better." *Openness to experience* appeared to be a valid predictor of training proficiency and was also noted to be correlated with cognitive ability. *Extraversion* similarly appeared to be correlated with training proficiency. *Agreeableness* appeared not to predict job performance in any important way.

If some of these factors are to be sought in staff selection, it remains an open question as to whether the best way to assess them in relation of job performance is by psychological testing or by other means.

Reference Checks

After the employment interview, the use of reference checks is the next most common staff selection technique in current practice. It thus needs careful examination in the quest to improve staff selection. There is, however, a paucity of current research literature on the subject. A comprehensive review of the literature on reference checks was undertaken in 1979 by Muchinsky. He found that with one exception, studies of the reliability and validity of reference checks yielded extremely low correlations with criterion measures. Problems of leniency and restriction of range seem to be inevitable. Not surprisingly, supervisors' references were more valid than personal references, but even these yielded poor results.

Muchinsky (1979) noted also that there was a problem with the validity of criterion measures, but that the main problem was clearly with the reference itself. One study reviewed by Muchinsky (Carrol & Nash, 1972, cited in Muchinsky) yielded different results. Using a specifically designed, structured, forced-choice question reference, the researchers produced a relatively high correlation of 0.64 between reference checks and performance ratings. In his conclusions, Muchinsky recommends that references be used to screen out unsuitable candidates rather than to rank suitable candidates. A second recommendation is:

> Rather than continually pleading for additional routine validation research, perhaps what would be more beneficial would be a greater emphasis on innovations involving the development of new design techniques . . . Perhaps the amount of incremental validity that reference reports provide for employer selection decisions can be enhanced through the investigation of different means of collecting and reporting the information they provide. (p. 296)

In a more recent review of the reference report, or reference check, Dobson (1989) concludes similarly that current research suggests that references are not valid as predictors of future job success.

> Consequently, one cannot recommend the use of the typical reference report in selection . . . There is little doubt that, potentially, reference reports are an extremely valuable selection method. Of course, the problem is how to obtain the information from the referee in a reliable and error-free manner, and how to ensure that it is valid to the prediction of job success. (p. 466)

Dobson goes on to provide some of the answers to this question. They include favoring oral over written references, basing questions on job analysis, providing as much structure as possible, using various measures to make the information received as behaviorally-based as possible, avoiding rating scales, providing the referee with some relevant background information about the job, obtaining a number of references on each applicant, and assessing the reference in the light of other information available on the applicant.

The approaches suggested by Muchinsky in 1979 and Dobson 10 years later parallel the way forward suggested by research on the employment interview, namely, the progressive move towards more structured formats.

While not approaching the degree of structure utilized in the Carroll and Nash study, two texts on personnel selection (Dessler, 1988; Pecora and Austin, 1987) do provide some ideas for standardizing reference checks. At a very minimum, it would seem desirable for child welfare agencies to design structured *pro formas* along these lines.

The question of written versus verbal references needs to be addressed. Unlike the United Kingdom and the United States, in residential child care in Australia references are usually done by telephone. Applicants may offer written references, which are usually written specifically for each job application. However, a letter of reference is unlikely to be other than positive and evaluating the objectivity of the referee is even more difficult with a written reference than one taken by telephone.

In commenting on various selection methods, Guion (1989) states:

> I suspect . . . that any improvement made in the use of references will come about by treating the reference check as a structured interview, albeit by telephone; I hold little hope for written references. Reliance on the integrity, motivation, knowledge, and willingness of letter writers seems so doomed as to merit no comment. (p. 124)

There are some arguments for trying to implement written references, such as the chance to send a structured form to be completed. However, experience would suggest that this is likely to lead to a poor response (Dobson, 1989). It would appear then, that the major focus of practice improvement should be the telephone reference. Guion says that the same methods leading to more valid interviews, such as job analysis, structured and job-related questioning, and training of staff in making judgements, are likely to lead to improved telephone reference checks.

Another problem with references is that they are generally selected by the applicant, who is likely to select out any negative ones. Murray (1986) claims that with signed authorization, employers can feel free to contact all potential referees and former employers regarding the applicant's character and work history and are not restricted to checking references listed on the application form. However, applicants should be put on notice that the employer plans to do this.

The competence of the referees themselves also needs to be considered. Loretto (1986) comments that references, whether oral or written, are extremely unreliable unless the source is personally known to the manager to be trustworthy and competent to judge. These standards are not easily fulfilled.

Legal issues around reference checks pertain to errors in the way reference checks are carried out and in the negligence implied by not doing them at all. Background verification, or reference checking, is a technique that may contribute to discrimination (Equal Employment Opportunity Commission, 1978) and is the reason that some employers now refuse to give reference material apart from basic information, such as confirming dates of employment (Dessler, 1988; Dobson, 1989). On the other hand, several cases of negligent hire in the United States, where an employee later caused damage to another party, have been won, in part or in full, because of the failure to check appropriate references (Besnoff, 1989).

Residential child care and the reference check

Peters and Getz (1986) stress the importance of the reference for the selection of child care workers and recommend that the most useful references are ones that specify the qualifications of the observer, indicate the duration of acquaintance and the situations under which the observations took place, provide judgments as to the personal characteristics, level of commitment, and special skills of the applicant, and rank the individual in comparison with others.

The Warner Report (United Kingdom Department of Health, 1992) takes a clear position that any legal issues must be considered in the light of the overwhelming duty of care to the children and young people in the care of a children's home. The legal liability for references must be recognized, and the person giving the reference must ensure that it is neither inaccurate nor omits any relevant material on the suitability of the applicant for the post. The reference must not be defamatory; however, if it is given with due care and without malice, the referee has the defence of "qualified privilege" against any defamation action by an applicant. Alternatively, if it omits relevant information, a new employer who suffers resulting damages may have a cause of action against the referee.

Other Assessment Methods

Given the problems of validity associated with employment interviews and reference checks, there have been some moves to establish alternative selection methods, usually as additions to conventional practice rather than substitutes. There appears to be limited research on these practices; most articles report on small field trials of innovative methods.

Hanson and Balestreri-Spiro (1985) outline the function of the Assessment Center, which provides a range of alternative methods of selection such as written exercises, oral presentations, and the "in-basket" method. With such methods, he claims that good applicants who do not interview well can be identified, saving the employer the cost of missing good candidates and having to re-recruit. The use of assessment centers is expensive, and some authorities (Dessler, 1988; Fletcher, personal communication, 1994) suggest that it may be possible to obtain equally good results with simpler and more cost-efficient selection methods.

Denholm (1988) describes a range of methods, in addition to the interview, used in hiring school-based youth workers, including written assignments, behavioral vignettes in various forms, and brief work tests. Honig (1979), writing about the selection of day care staff, advocates a three-part process, including an interview, a role-play, and observation, with twenty questions to be answered afterwards. Writing specifically about residential child care, Peters and Getz (1986) recommend the use of on-site observation of work skills where possible.

In relation to residential child care, Warner (cited in United Kingdom Department of Health, 1992) advocates monitored visits to children's homes, written exercises, and possibly group exercises, aptitude tests, and personality profiling for senior staff.

LEGAL AND ETHICAL ISSUES

Most of the available literature on legal and ethical issues in personnel selection is in the United States. This literature provides some useful guidelines that may be applied in general terms to caregiver selection.

The United States Equal Employment Opportunity Commission (EEOC) and the American Psychological Association (1980) provide detailed standards for the personnel selection process, including ethical standards. Nevertheless, London and Bray (1980) comment that standards do not exist for all situations, and that "standards are often ambiguous, contrary and far from intuitively obvious."

Negligent Hire

"Negligent hire" is a legal term used when a party takes court action claiming damages as a result of poor employment practices. The issue of negligent hire litigation is a field of growing concern in the United States.

> In the past, such cases were typically brought by employees who were either not hired, not promoted, or discharged. New negligent hire actions are increasingly being instituted by innocent third parties, such as customers who have been injured by the criminal, violent or negligent acts of an employee. (Besnoff, 1989, p. 11)

This issue has been addressed in relation to the field of day care in an article by Murray (1986):

> All of the negligent hire cases stress the awareness of the opportunity for crime created by the circumstances of the employment and impose a higher duty of care in the investigation process when the risk is greater. Child care center directors are now quite aware that the potential for crime exists in a child care center and, indeed, it is difficult to imagine a population at a higher risk of harm than young children who are under the complete control of the adults who attend them. Consequently, in litigation, it is likely that courts

> will impose a very stringent duty of investigation upon child care center employers. (p. 28)

Murray's comments about the special circumstances pertaining to day child care are equally relevant to residential child care.

Negligent hire is not yet an important issue in Australia, but the lack of attention to personnel selection practices and increasing media attention to abuse in care means that it is potentially so. As in many other areas of practice which arguably should have been addressed for ethical and professional reasons, the issues of competent carer selection may finally be addressed through the fear of litigation.

Equal Employment Opportunity (EEO)

Equality employment opportunity (EEO): The American context. As discussed earlier, much attention in selection research in the United States has been directed towards questions of equal employment opportunity and the issue of adverse effect on minority groupings.

The *Uniform Guidelines on Employee Selection Procedures* (Equal Employment Opportunity Commission [EEOC], 1978) outlines the legal requirements for the validation of selection procedures in the United States. It is interesting to note, however, that the selection interview was an issue in less than 1% of the more than 8000 EEO cases in the United States courts reported between 1979-1987, according to Campion and Arvey (1989). Perhaps because of this, many American employers have turned away from the use of selection tests back to the interview.

Dessler (1988) makes the point that asking questions concerning race, religion, age, sex, or national origin are not illegal per se under United States federal laws. However, they are viewed with disfavor by the EEOC, and the burden of proof will always be on the employer to prove that they are both related to success or failure on the job and not unfairly discriminatory. This could be a difficult case to argue. Murray (1986) and Pecora and Austin (1987) detail examples of questions to ask applicants which are either acceptable or not regarding apparent EEO intent.

Campion and Arvey (1989) examined United States federal and state court decisions that included the employment interview as a fair employment practice issue. The interview was most often referred to in sex (47%) and race (31%) discrimination suits, followed by age (12%). Employers were criticized for the inappropriate racial and/or gender mix of the interviewing team, insufficient training and experience of the interviewing team in the hiring process, not providing formal instructions to interviewers, the inadequacy of interviewer training, the inappropriateness of an interviewing format that had not been reviewed for many years, inadequate record-keeping of interview notes and decisions, a lack of identification of qualifications and criteria being used, and inappropriate interviewer questions such as questions relating to marital and parental status, handicaps, and conviction records.

Campion and Arvey (1989) recommend that employers:

1. develop job descriptions;
2. implement selection and training of interviewers;
3. use appropriate questioning techniques, including job relevancy, and that the same questions should be asked of all applicants;
4. introduce review to counter subjectivity arguments, for example, multiple interviewers or panel interviews, and use management committees to review interviewer findings and recommendations;
5. keep records for several years;
6. monitor for disparate impact. (pp. 66-67)

The American Psychological Association (1980) comments on the obligation to consider, as far as possible, the possibility of bias or other contamination.

> There is no clear path to truth in these matters. A criterion difference between older and younger employees, or day or night shift may reflect bias in raters, equipment or conditions, or it may reflect genuine differences in performance. What is required is the anticipation and reduction of the possibility of bias, alertness to this possibility, protection against it insofar as is feasible, and use of the best judgment possible in evaluating the data. (p. 7)

A further concern is the right of the employee to be protected, as far as possible, from personnel selection mistakes. Since there is no foolproof selection method, mistakes are inevitable. Reasonable opportunities should be given for review and reconsideration when possible, while preserving the security of procedures (EEOC, 1976).

London and Bray (1980) say that, in general, personnel decisions should be closely monitored to be sure they are fair and conform to professional and legal standards, and for this reason it is important that they are well documented.

EEO: The Australian context. Five acts of Parliament have particular relevance to the application of EEO in personnel selection in Victoria. These are:

- The Victorian Equal Opportunity Act (Victoria, 1995);
- The Disability Discrimination Act (Australia, 1992);
- The Sex Discrimination Act (Australia, 1984);
- The Racial Discrimination Act (Australia, 1975);
- The Human Rights and Equal Opportunity Commission Act (Australia, 1986).

With some areas of overlap between them, these Acts together prohibit discrimination in employment on the basis of gender, sexual preference, marital status, pregnancy, parental status, race, religious or political beliefs, or disability (actual or assumed). Further, it is unlawful for an employer to discriminate against a person because of an impairment if they are the best-qualified person for the job and can perform adequately the required duties (Commissioner for Equal Opportunity, 1992a).

Some exceptions and exemptions are available to specified employers for specific reasons in the *General Statutory Exemptions* (Commissioner for Equal Opportunity, 1992b, pp. 108-110). In residential child care, these include sex and marital status discrimination. Most complaints to the Victorian Equal Opportunity Commission in 1991-1992 were on the basis of sex discrimination, and these were overwhelmingly in the area of employment (Commission for Equal Opportunity, 1992).

In residential child care, issues of discrimination may arise particularly in relation to gender, but as mentioned earlier, such discrimination is likely to favor women, as the evidence is that there is bias against men when a job is regarded as stereotypically female (Campion & Arvey, 1989). In addition to the problem of gender stereotyping being used to discriminate against men, the more difficult issue arises from the fact that almost all sexual abusers of children are male (Community Services Commission, 1996). Research suggests that while some profiles of the sex offender exist, none of these are definitive, and many pedophiles are clever people who present with the responses of a highly competent child care worker (Moriarty, 1990). They are also very resourceful in gaining access to children via their employment (Lanning, 1986) and tend to seek employment in child care centers as teachers or counsellors (Moriarty, 1990). An extreme point of view regarding the pedophile issue is advocated by Pringle (1993), who says that men should not be permitted to work in residential child care.

Therefore, EEO considerations require that selection practice in the area of residential care be as thorough and stringent as possible if discrimination is not to occur through fear of selecting unsuitable or abusive applicants.

Privacy and freedom of information

The right of applicants to privacy and confidentiality includes their right of access to information obtained about them and their right to give informed consent. Various tensions exist between these rights and the rights and needs of the employer to obtain valid information upon which to make personnel decisions. As indicated above, a good deal of controversy exists around the ethics of personnel testing in personnel selection. London and Bray (1980) recommend that employees and applicants not be required or pressured to take a personality test or any other examination that constitutes, in their opinion, an invasion of privacy, regardless of the test's validity (p. 894). Others take the further position that asking the applicant to reveal details of thought or emotion not relevant to job performance is an invasion of privacy. London and Bray conclude that such views need to be balanced against the value to the organization, society and individuals themselves of accurate employment decisions.

Confidentiality appears to be a clearer area. London and Bray (1980) cite the *American Psychological Association Ethical Standards of Psychologists* (1977) to the effect that confidentiality may only be breached when there is a clear and imminent danger to an individual or society and then only to appropriate professional workers or public authorities. The "right to know" test result is generally becoming more respected and operationalized in the United States; however, it has to be weighed against the need to maintain the security of test items in order to maintain their validity

Another complex issue regarding the right to know relates to referees' reports or letters of recommendation. "Here as in other areas, there is a conflict between the rights of the individual and the validity of the information obtained. An important research question is whether those named as references will supply negative information if they know the applicant will have access to it" (London & Bray, 1980, p. 896).

One option for dealing with this dilemma follows a model established in the arena of education by the United States Congress in 1974, giving students the right to inspect their records. "Now students choose whether or not to waive this right before asking someone to complete a recommendation form. [This]. . . may be a viable solution to employee complaints about confidential information they believe may be used against them" (London & Bray, 1980, p. 896).

The right to know also applies to the right of an individual to be told every potential use of test results.

The lack of Australian literature on the subject suggests that the area of privacy and freedom of information in staff recruitment may be less clearly defined in this country.

Ethics and Validation Studies

The validation of personnel selection procedures is an extremely difficult and complex process requiring for best results an investment of time and resources that is not always practical. There is, however, an expectation that those who develop personnel selection procedures collect evidence to show a relationship between decisions based on assessments made by that procedure and criteria such as job performance or other pertinent job behavior such as training performance or advancement (American Psychological Association, 1980, p. 1). In this context, a poor study is not seen as better than none, and that if a criterion-related study is not possible, alternative methods of validation such as content validity may be chosen. The United States government is also beginning to acknowledge that this may be desirable (London & Bray, 1980, p. 900).

Where the persons developing personnel selection methods are not psychologists, a supervising psychologist should be responsible for ensuring that appropriate standards are met. This would include training, monitoring, and ongoing research into the accuracy and appropriateness of the procedure. The psychologist must clarify with the employer what can be expected from the types of test or assessment development and validation which the employer is willing to fund.

The question of validation of selection procedures is particularly difficult in situations where small organizations with limited budgets are charged with the responsibility of developing fair and valid selection procedures. One approach to this dilemma may be to draw on best known practice from scientifically-validated research, with appropriate allowances for the particular employment situation.

RECRUITMENT AND SELECTION IN RESIDENTIAL CHILD CARE

The United States: The Question of Psychological Testing Again

In the United States, research interest in personnel selection practices is increasing in the field of residential child care. The difficulty of making objective and valid assessments of applicants' abilities is a challenging one in this field because the actual job performance appears to be very dependent upon personal skills and qualities. The common thread running through the American studies is an attempt to develop a standardized "test" of personality or performance based on personal qualities and skills. Despite the controversy around the use of personality testing in staff selection discussed earlier, a *prima facie* argument could be made that, if the personality characteristics of effective residential child care workers are understood, personality testing may become a relevant way of assessing potential job performance.

Unfortunately, the various attempts to come to grips with this issue have led different researchers in different directions, and there has been little replication of previous studies. A relatively early review of work in this area was conducted by Saunders and Pappanikou (1970) who concluded that, "Little progress has been made in the area of psychometric selection of child care workers" (p. 20). Colligan, Goke and Endres (1977) identified a number of studies used to establish psychological tests such as the Rorschach, the California Personality Inventory, the Minnesota Multiphasic Personality Inventory, the Thematic Apperception Test, and others.

They concluded that small sample sizes were a major limitation in almost all of the earlier studies. Colligan, Goke and Endres (1977) studied 23 employed residential child care workers whose results on a battery of psychological tests were correlated with supervisors' ratings. Results seemed to be promising but required further cross-validation, and plans were underway for a larger study for this purpose. Such a study has not been published. Similarly, Schaefer studied 14 residential child care staff in which self-assessment on an adjective checklist was measured against a perceived ideal type. Again, results appeared promising and plans were made for a larger study.

The next systematic approach to the question of validating employment interviews for residential child care workers was made by Maloney et al. (1983) in North Carolina. This was a very small study of 11 couples in which behavioral vignettes were used as test materials. Applicants' responses to these vignettes or stimulus situations were rated on a 7-point Likert scale. In addition, interview performance was rated on a series of 7-point Likert scales. The high performance applicants scored significantly higher on the behavioral vignettes than the low-performance applicants but not on interview performance. The study does not, however, detail the nature of the interview (for example, structured or unstructured).

Mufson (1986) used the California Psychological Inventory (Megargee, 1972) to determine whether a high-functioning group of child care workers would display different characteristics than a low-functioning group. The two groups did reveal significant differences on 7 of the 18 scales of the test. High scores on scales measuring Dominance, Capacity for Status, Sociability, Social Presence, Self-Acceptance, and Tolerance appeared to be associated with high performance. In addition, low Femininity–a scale measuring more than traditional gender distinctions–appeared to be associated with high performance. Mufson's total sample was 45; the final sample was 28.

A much larger study of personnel selection for residential child care workers has been undertaken by Ross and Hoeltke (1985; 1987). Over 100 subjects were engaged in a longitudinal study of an interviewing tool called the Child Care Perceiver (Selection Research Inc., 1982) for the selection of residential child care workers. The method is based upon the hypothetical construct of Life Themes that are said to characterize individuals who have the capacity to perform highly in specific fields. The Life Themes of a specific occupational group are identified by studying high performers in that particular field.

The Life Themes identified for high performing residential child care workers, each described in some detail, were Mission, Relationship, Empathy, Responsibility, Kinesthetic/Work Orientation, Gestalt, Activation, Courage, Objectivity, and Developer. The results claimed for the Perceiver seem impressive. It yielded significant correlations against self-ratings, supervisors' ratings, child resident ratings, and institutional climate. A study for EEO acceptability revealed that it seemed to be free of bias for age, race, and gender.

Another large study (n = 270) was undertaken around the same time by Wasmund and Tate (1988) that explored the discriminant properties of the Sixteen Personality Factor Questionnaire (Cattel, Eber, & Tatsuoka, 1980) in discerning the personality characteristics of high-functioning versus low-functioning residential child care workers. Five of the 16 factors were found to differentiate most from least effective child care workers. These were Warmth, Intelligence, Assertiveness, Social Reservation, and Conservatism. In addition, very effective workers scored lower on Boldness than less effective workers.

These characteristics seem to have some similarities to those identified by Mufson (1986), although the overall constellation of personality factors predicted high performance correctly only 70% of the time. This may relate in part to the unreliability of the supervisors' ratings used as the criterion variable. Another more general concern about this study is that, according to Walsh (cited in Buros, 1978), the Sixteen Personality Factor Questionnaire is a failure and impossible to recommend for any use from the most basic research to the most programatically-oriented applications.

Moriarty (1990) addressed the more specific question of how to screen out pedophiles and child abusers. He suggested investigating the utility of two other tests: the Personnel Selection Inventory (PSI) and the Child Abuse Inventory. However, studies of the Child Abuse Inventory indicated that it is unsuitable for the screening of residential child care workers. The PSI is yet another tool for predicting behaviors of residential child care workers, designed by London House, Inc., in Illinois, a management consultancy firm specializing in staff selection. Jones, Joy and Martin (1990) recommend that the PSI be used with other credible selection devices such as interviews, reference checks, and effective monitoring programs. The validation studies of the PSI documented by Jones and Joy (1987) and Jones, Joy, and Martin (1990) are encouraging, but they are small and criterion variables themselves suffer from the usual difficulties of validity.

In a student paper, Burgess (n.d.) has reviewed many of the above studies with a view to finding tools for the assessment of applicants for studies in child and youth care counselling. He points to the continuing concern with "false positives," that is, those applicants who appear in interview to be likely to have talent but do not do well subsequently, and suggests that a fruitful area for further research may be to interview in some detail both students who have been unsuccessful in the job and those who were screened out in order to establish if common patterns of life themes exist in this group.

Herman (1993) reviewed some of the available scales for measuring behaviors and personality characteristics that may be detrimental to child and youth care work for the purpose of enhancing the screening of volunteers for the Big Brothers, Big Sisters program. Herman notes the lack of reliability and/or validity of each scale.

On a more general approach to recruitment and selection in residential child care, Peters and Getz (1986) recommended, among other things, recognition of the value of different personal approaches to the delivery of residential care rather than one fixed model, an inclusive approach to short-listing for interviews, and the use of on-site observation of work skills where possible.

Overall, the theme in the research on residential staff selection is the search for more structured and valid approaches by using a range of different test materials. Results have, however, been disappointing, and no general standard has emerged, according to Stuck (personal communication, 1994).

Developments in the United Kingdom

Prior to 1992, only one British publication was found that focused specifically on residential child care staff selection. Kahan, Banner, and Lane (1986) wrote a booklet for the Social Care Association on the selection of residential carers, outlining broad general guidelines regarding good practice in the recruitment and retention of residential child care workers. This booklet recommended, among other standard good practice, consideration of extended visits or involvement in a residential unit, including young people in the experience, as a two-way assessment process.

More recent concern in the United Kingdom about residential child care staff selection has emanated from a series of scandals about abuse in children's homes and in 1992 led to a committee of inquiry into the selection, development, and management of staff in children's homes. The report of this inquiry (United Kingdom Department of Health, 1992) advocated the use of a range of selection devices in addition to the selection interview. A controversial recommendation was the mandatory use of psychological tests for senior positions and their optional use for direct care positions.

Surprisingly, the report did not draw on current research on the employment interview and made no recommendations regarding the structuring of the selection interview. It did, however, recommend the use of alternative staff selection methods such as visits to the homes (informally involving children in care), written exercises, group exercises, and thorough reference checking in addition to the careful use of conventional methods.

The Warner Inquiry in turn led to the establishment of the Support Force for Children's Residential Care (194; 1995a; 1995b), a body that spent two years working on a range of areas of good practice. Central to its work was a role in furthering good practice in the recruitment, selection, and management of staff in children's homes. The Support Force subsequently published a *Recruitment and Selection Techniques: Database* (1994) and a *Code of Practice for the Employment of Residential Child Care Workers* (1995a), a practical manual that included a section outlining briefly some recommended methods for staff selection. This manual followed the recommendations of the Warner Report about selection processes. A subsequent publication of the Support Force in the same year, *Good Care Matters* (1995b), addresses broader issues of ensuring quality residential child care, including behavior management, involving young people, complaints mechanisms, and abuse prevention.

In a subsequent recent research study on the characteristics of good residential child care staff in Cleveland, the United Kingdom, a sample of 25 residential social workers (i.e., residential child care workers) who were identified as good performers were interviewed about recent events in their child care experience, and the behavior patterns were described and analyzed by Robinson and King (1996; McMillan, Robinson, & King, n.d.). Nine groups of specific behaviors were described that were said to characterize the most effective residential workers. These nine groups are Behavioral Analysis, Empathy, Nurturing, Developing Young People, Positive Confrontation, Self-Control, Openness, Perseverance, and Positive Attitude. Some consistency was noted between these findings and those cited above of Ross and Hoeltke (1985; 1987) and Wasmund and Tate (1988).

Involving young people in staff selection

Other innovative work that has emerged from the United Kingdom in recent years describes the process of involving young people in and from care in the selection of staff.

Lindsay and Rayner (1993) involved a group of young adults who had lived in care in the process of selecting persons for appointment to an Independent Persons Project, and on the basis of this experience called for more consideration of this process in recruiting residential care staff. These young people conducted their interviews in collaboration with staff but without staff in the interview room. These authors also suggested that this process may have a deterrent effect on applicants who do not wish to work in partnership with young people, or worse, who have ulterior motives for seeking such work.

Berridge and Wenman (1995) worked with a group of young people (ages 15-16) living in a children's home to involve them in the selection of a research worker. This worker was to spend some time living in a number of children's homes in order to study their programs. Staff were present for the interviews conducted by the young people. These authors also advocated this process to be explored in residential child care staff selection. The United Kingdom Save the Children Fund has also recently been working on in-house policy documents regarding procedures for the involvement of young people in the selection of program staff (United Kingdom Save the Children Fund, 1996). The SCV policy on involving young people is written from a strong children's rights perspective, echoing international obligations under the UN Convention on the Rights of the Child, Article 12 (United Nations General Assembly, 1989).

Developments in Australia

Interest in the subject of residential child care staff selection in Australia has, until very recently, been to a large extent peripheral to broader concerns about residential care standards and practice. These broader concerns have been expressed in a series of review reports (Buzatu, 1987; Department of Community Welfare Service, 1985; Phillip Institute of Technology, 1982; South Australia Community Welfare Advisory Committee, 1973).

Despite repeated calls in these reports for improvement in staff selection in residential child care, the literature review did not reveal any published Australian material specifically on this topic prior to the commencement of this research project.

Since the commencement of this study, the context of this inquiry changed considerably. Interest in the topic in Australia has increased considerably, largely as a result of public awareness and media interest in the discovery that abuse in care has been widespread in some quarters here as it has overseas. Some training in this field has now taken place as a result of this research project. Published material on the topic is detailed below but remains limited.

As mentioned in the Introduction, this research study and the model of staff selection it generated has also led to the writing of two field handbooks. The first is *Recruiting and Selecting Residential Care Workers* (Kildonan Child and Family Services, 1999). *Choose with Care: A Recruitment Guide for Organizations Working with Children* is available as part of this volume. Also based on the work of this study is an article on the topic of avoiding recruiting a pedophile into child and youth care (Kiraly, 1996). It advocates a range of good practice measures in staff selection, together with a series of deterrent measures.

In 1995, the NSW Community Services Commission undertook an inquiry into recruitment, screening, and appointment practices in funded welfare services for children, the aged, and the disabled in NSW, and subsequently published a report entitled *Who Cares? Protecting People in Residential Care* (Community Services Commission, 1996). The report recommended a package of staff selection processes to include suitable training for managers engaged in staff selection, an adequate information package for applicants, including a program description, a job description, person specification, a code of conduct, and a notice of the declarations, authorizations, consents, and fingerprints which may be required; and some suggestions for improved methods of selection.

Criminal Records Checks and Residential Child Care

Criminal records checks are becoming a routine requirement for residential child care staff and child welfare personnel in the United States, the United Kingdom, and in Australia. In Victoria, they became general practice from about 1989. Some words of caution about their use are made in the literature, however. Warner (United Kingdom Department of Health, 1992) cautions against their use in lieu of thorough selection practices. Carter (1986) makes the same case much more forcefully. She argues that criminal history check requirements have led to a lowering of standards of entry to the field of child care in the United States by providing an implied standard that if the applicant does not have a criminal record, the person will meet the minimum qualifications to work with children. Moriarty (1990) highlights the fact that less than 1% of people who engage in acts of child molestation have a criminal record. Warner cites figures suggesting that "an estimated 4% of all offences committed result in a criminal conviction, so police checks are going to reveal only a very small proportion of child abusers" (United Kingdom Department of Health, 1992, p. 72). It is thus likely that the only benefit of a criminal records check is that it may avoid a rare catastrophic mistake in staff selection, and possibly provide some deterrent effect.

Hebenton and Thomas (1989; 1992: 1994a; 1994b) sound a cautionary note about the rapid rise in the United Kingdom of criminal records checks and some ensuing poor practice, including lack of confidentiality, checking on a number of applicants rather than only the preferred applicant, checking on people applying for jobs that do not warrant a check, police disclosure of information with the status of gossip as well as convictions, lack of opportunity for individuals to comment on their alleged record, and lack of clear guidelines as to which offences constitute grounds for rejection for a particular position. Hebenton and Thomas thus propose that it is important to have satisfactory processes in place to look after the civil rights of people undergoing criminal records checks. This includes clear guidelines as to what convictions might warrant rejection for a position.

ISSUES RELATING TO METHODOLOGY

The overwhelming issue in personnel selection research is to demonstrate that particular selection methods are valid, in that they can be shown to measure and predict accurately future performance of successful candidates for the job in question. "The costs of time and money and the limited number of people about whom the same type of decision is made make a predictive or concurrent validity study impractical in many situations" (London and Bray, 1980, p. 900). There are, in fact, a number of reasons why it is particularly difficult to demonstrate the validity of a particular selection method. These will be dealt with in turn.

The Problem of the Criterion Variable

As mentioned elsewhere in this literature review, a major problem in validation of staff selection procedures is that of finding a valid criterion variable. The variable most often used is the performance rating of a supervisor. This is a notoriously unreliable criterion (Meyer, 1987; Fletcher, 1992). Smith (1991) comments, ". . . no criterion of success is perfect. Many studies use opinions of supervisors . . . It is like calibrating a new thermometer against an 18th-century thermometer that is only 80% accurate: the new one can never appear to be more than 80% accurate" (p. 41). When combining the error in the criterion measure with the unavoidable error in the selection process, it is clear why results are at times disappointing.

Measures of performance appraisal, an ostensibly more sophisticated way of rating staff performance, are plagued with the same errors. A number of studies have attempted to train appraisers to eliminate rater error, with very limited success (Bernardin & Buckley, 1981; Bernardin & Pence, 1980). Over time, it was realized that many of these programs simply taught raters to substitute one form of rater error (leniency) with another (severity) and ignored the real issue of accuracy. The main cause of rater inaccuracy seemed to be the perceived fear of the rater that accurate, unfavorable ratings will damage the relationship between the appraiser and appraisee. Fletcher (1992), a leading authority on performance appraisal, holds little faith in the accuracy of behaviorally-based, quantitative performance appraisal systems, and maintains that most managers are unable to rate accurately except to perceive extremes of "good" and "bad" performance.

Other criterion variables have been utilized at times. Meyer (1987), in an attempt to move away from supervisor ratings, used promotional progress in his commercial sector study. This would be a criterion of limited relevance to residential child care, as promotional opportunities are particularly limited in this field. Maloney et al. (1983), in a small study of residential child care workers, used a range of on-the-job performance measures taken from the regular consumer evaluation conducted in the program. Seven consumer groups–resident youths, their parents, teachers, juvenile court and social service personnel, community board members and program directors–all took part in the evaluation of staff performance. The Total Evaluation Score was based upon the average of scores from all seven consumer groups.

Ross and Hoeltke's (1985; 1987) larger United States research project in residential child care staff selection used four measures as criterion variables: self-rating, supervisor's rating, residents' rating, and institutional climate. While these studies offer the possibility that a broader range of criterion variables may improve validity, there is still little means of determining the accuracy of these additional criterion variables. A further problem is that considerable additional funding needs to be available for a study of a statistically significant size if a range of criterion variables are to be adopted. The issue of the criterion variable raises substantial concerns for a further attempt to determine best practice in residential child care staff selection by quantitative methods, particularly with limited resources.

Type 1 and Type 2 Errors

While the validation of personnel selection methods by the use of a criterion variable such as supervisors' ratings is an apparently reasonable method, it does not address the question of whether potentially competent staff have been selected out in the interview process (Type 2 error). Type 2 errors are, of course, even more difficult to detect than Type 1 errors (false positive selection decisions), as the possibly competent individuals selected out are lost to the research study.

Rowe (1989) says that interviewers seem to be more interested in collecting unfavorable information than favorable information, and that the unfavorable information has a greater impact upon selection decisions. This phenomenon would seem to be related to the concern of interviewers that a "false positive" selection (Type 1 error), may have serious consequences for the decision-maker, while the other error, that of rejecting good candidates (Type 2 error), is likely to go undetected. Rowe also noted the resistance of interviewers to altering this bias, even when experimental conditions appeared to make such a change favorable.

Peters and Getz (1986) suggestion to be very inclusive in listing the maximum number of candidates for interviewing may be one way to minimize Type 2 errors; beyond this, the challenge seems to be to influence interviewers to pay more attention to positive information.

This raises the issue of how the short-listing process is done, as well as of how to try to minimize the screening out of competent staff in selection processes. In a field where managers often struggle to find sufficient skilled staff, this needs to be addressed as part of improving staff selection.

Other Issues of Research Design

The scientific study of staff selection methods also has some other problems. First, few employers are in the position of recruiting at one time sufficient employees to become the subjects of a validation study, even if resources were available to complete a study of a statistically significant size. A further complication is that, as mentioned above, those applicants who are rejected are not available for validation of their job performance. Many studies, therefore, have resorted to some form of simulation in the academic environment using student interviewers and/or job applicants, particularly when exploring specific interview effects, for example, dress and impression management strategies (Kacmar, Ratcliff, & Ferris, 1989, p. 40). Results from such studies need to be regarded with caution (Weitzel, 1989) as to whether they can be regarded as transferable to real life situations.

The difficulty of replicating a tightly structured interview was shown by Latham and Saari (1984), who gained invalid results in one experiment, only later discovering that instructions were not followed exactly. The necessity for the research worker then to be present when the data is being collected is thus highlighted–a large assignment.

SUMMARY

There is a wealth of personnel selection research knowledge that has yet to be applied fully to personnel practice. Further, it is clear that no one personnel selection method has proved to be ultimately successful on its own. Current practice in residential child care staff selection is also not well-informed by knowledge in personnel selection research, and it is not clear which personnel selection processes are most appropriate to this field.

The body of scientific research on residential child care staff selection per se is small, largely exploratory, and has yielded no clear direction for professional practice. Much of this research relates to explorations of psychological testing in carer selection; overall, outcomes in this area have proved disappointing.

There is scattered information in the literature which is suggestive of the characteristics of a skilled residential child care worker, but no clear overall picture. There are significant problems in establishing a valid quantitative research process for measuring the effectiveness of particular methods of staff selection in a field setting. These difficulties include problems in establishing reliable criterion variables, the unavailability of unsuccessful job applicants to the research process, and resource constraints affecting pragmatics of sample size and time frames over which job performance could be measured.

Chapter 3

Methodology

The research questions were:

> Question 1: What are the principles of quality residential care?
>
> Question 2: How can the process of recruitment and selection provide the best chance of obtaining skilled residential child care staff?
>
> Question 2a: What are the characteristics of a skilled residential child care worker?
>
> Question 2b: What are the features and components of a good staff selection package?
>
> Question 3: Is it in the interests of the resident children that the birth children of staff live in a family group home?

A NATURALISTIC AND QUALITATIVE METHODOLOGY

> Qualitative inquiry cultivates the most useful of all human capacities–the capacity to learn from others. (Patton, 1990, p. 7)

Several factors led to the development of the methodology. The first was that the literature review pointed to a real difficulty in establishing a reliable and valid criterion variable against which to evaluate a model of staff selection. Both supervisory ratings and quantitative performance appraisal ratings in general have been found to be very unsatisfactory for this purpose. Alternative criteria such as promotional progress, ratings by other parties, and organizational climate indices are either inap-

[Haworth co-indexing entry note]: "Methodology." Kiraly, Meredith. Co-published simultaneously in *Child & Youth Services* (The Haworth Press, Inc.) Vol. 23, No. 1/2, 2001, pp. 51-57; and: *Residential Child Care Staff Selection: Choose with Care* (Meredith Kiraly) The Haworth Press, Inc., 2001, pp. 51-57. Single or multiple copies of this article are available for a fee from The Haworth Document Delivery Service [1-800-HAWORTH 9:00 a.m. - 5:00 p.m. (EST). E-mail address: getinfo@haworthpressinc.com].

propriate to the context or are not themselves clearly identified as reliable and valid measures of job performance. Patton (1990) states that:

> Another reason for using qualitative methods is that for a particular outcome no acceptable, valid and reliable quantitative measures exist. . . . Where outcome measurements have not been developed and tested, it is more appropriate to gather descriptive information about what happens as a result of program activities than to use some scale that has the merit of being quantitative but whose validity and reliability are suspect. (p. 130)

Another consideration was that it seemed that it might be beneficial to obtain an in-depth understanding of what the various stakeholders in the staff selection process saw as the desirable attributes of a residential child care worker and important ways to improve the selection process.

A further consideration was the wish to understand the views of young people in care and their parents regarding the research questions. Berridge (1992b) has called for the perspective of young people in care to be explored in any research into residential care, and this concern has been echoed by the Victorian Association of Young People in Care [VAYPIC].

The best approach to gaining the information sought seemed thus to be an exploratory one, as the field of study was new and complex. However, it also seemed clear from the literature review that there was considerable relevant information available from the personnel selection field which needed to be explored in relation to its capacity to inform the residential child care field. The research plan thus needed to allow for the exploration of a field of ideas in some depth and breadth. Thus, the research methodology was designed to include a series of focus groups with all the relevant stakeholders.

By 1992, it was clear that significant activity was beginning to take place in the United Kingdom around the topic of residential child care staff selection. Communications were commenced with relevant authorities in the United Kingdom and the desirability of visiting the United Kingdom to learn from this work. This study tour was planned to explore current developments in the United Kingdom and elsewhere and to build on the literature review through discussions with some of the prominent writers on personnel selection and residential child care in the United Kingdom and the United States of America.

A further development in the methodology arose from the discovery of an article by Lindsay and Rayner (1993) on the involvement of young people in care in staff selection that was referred to me by Jim McAlinden, the Co-ordinator of the Victorian Association of Young People in Care (VAYPIC), during the recruitment of young people from VAYPIC for the focus groups. This material led to the development of questions about this topic for the focus groups. It also led to study tour interviews with the authors of the articles, young people involved in the process, and a child welfare research worker who underwent this selection method. As a result of this work, it was decided to trial this approach locally. Like the focus groups, it seemed that such a pilot project might also be an empowering way to engage young people in the research process.

The final shape of the overall methodology thus included the following three components:

- a series of eight focus groups,
- an international study tour,
- a pilot project involving young people and parents in staff selection.

AN ACTION RESEARCH METHODOLOGY

Kemmis and McTaggert (1988) describe action research as:

> . . . a form of *collective* self-reflective enquiry undertaken by participants in social situations in order to improve the rationality and justice of their own social or educational practices, as well as their understanding of these practices and the situations in which these practices are carried out. . . . The approach is only action research when it is *collaborative*, though it is important to realize that the action research of the group is achieved through the *critically examined action* of individual group members. . . . The linking of the terms "action" and "research" highlights the essential feature of the approach: trying out ideas in practice as a means of improvement and as a means of increasing knowledge. . . . Action research provides a way of working which links theory and practice into the one whole: ideas-in-action. (p. 5)

Kemmis and McTaggert (1988) describe the process of reflective inquiry, or analysis of data, as proceeding in a spiral of steps, each of which is composed of planning, action, and evaluation of the results of the action. Evaluation prepares for new action, sometimes modified on the basis of the first spiral of experience, or possibly going in a somewhat different direction. It is a flexible and responsive approach which encourages change in plans as people learn from experience. Modifications may need to be made at any stage. Group discussion is the vehicle for planning these changes and further action.

This model appeared to suit this project well. The research was undertaken by a collaborative process with the participants in each part of the project, and the learning from each part was logically applied to those following. A spiral of activity, reflection and modification, and further activity characterized the research process.

The research approach contained a strong emphasis on client empowerment. Both young people and parents expressed great satisfaction with being invited to participate in the focus groups and the pilot project, and they contributed rich and important insights. These experiences led to a heightened awareness of the value of listening to the perspective of young people and their families in the quest to improve residential child care.

As recommended by Patton (1990), in order for this naturalistic enquiry to be effective, "empathic neutrality," direct personal contact, and an active involvement in the research was required. I remained a practitioner in the residential child care field/child welfare field throughout the work. Some of the subjects in the focus groups were former clients, colleagues, and staff previously supervised. As a result of contact with past clients and colleagues, I needed to be willing to reciprocate their contribution with assistance according to their current needs. For example, in response to specific requests, I advocated within the welfare system on behalf of former clients and provided information to client and colleague participants. I provided feedback in the form of written reports to the members of the focus groups and to persons interviewed during the study tour. I wrote a reference for a young woman who assisted in staff selection, verifying her involvement and contribution to the selection process (which helped her to gain casual work).

COMPONENTS OF THE RESEARCH PROJECT

The Focus Groups

Eight focus groups were run in 1994, including a total of 76 subjects. The following groups were identified as the key stakeholders in the residential child care experience: young people who had been in care, parents of children in care, residential child care workers, and supervisors of residential workers. These people are the major stakeholders in the residential care experience and as such would be likely to be able to provide useful viewpoints from their differing perspectives. All of these were represented in the focus groups.

The focus groups addressed a series of topics relating to the recruitment, selection, and support of residential child care staff, and were designed to collect material that would contribute to answering the research questions.

Six groups were run in May, 1994: two of residential child care staff, two of young people who had been in care, one of parents who had had children in care, and one of supervisors.

Following this, there were three major sources of bias in the sample. First, most of the residential child care workers were workers from family group homes. Second, the parent's group had been screened for parents who had identified mental illnesses, intellectual disability, and chronic substance abuse, as they were seen to be less likely to function well in the large group setting. Nevertheless, parents with such disabilities make up a significant proportion of the parents of children in care, and as such it was seen as important to offer them an opportunity to be heard. Third, the parent's group was an all-female one. The few fathers who were able to be located and contacted were unable to be present on the day.

The first two biases were addressed by running two further groups, groups 7 and 8 in December of 1994. Group 7 consisted exclusively of rostered residential child care staff. Group 8 was a small group of parents with identified mental illnesses or intellectual disability. The final bias was not able to be addressed. Extensive searching failed to generate a group of fathers who were able and willing to attend the groups.

Apart from this group of men, participation rates were high. Few people dropped out, once committed. Each group yielded vigorous discussion and a wealth of creative ideas. Many participants expressed their satisfaction in being involved. In particular, both parents and young people expressed real appreciation of the opportunity to "have their say," as one parent put it. Despite the many traumas of their past, they proved able to reflect on their experiences with insight and an awareness of the difficult roles staff had to play in providing care to young people away from home. Staff were similarly appreciative of the opportunity, and eager to express their views.

The sessions were recorded and analyzed using methods recommended by Krueger (1988). A summary of responses to questions asked was made from the transcripts. A detailed report was also written and made available to participants, moderators, and other interested parties.

The Study Tour

The 7-week study tour was designed to allow for interviews with authorities in the field of personnel selection and residential child care/child welfare. The aim was to gain specific information relating to the research questions and other information on improving staffing and the delivery of quality care.

A number of key informants in personnel selection were identified from the literature, from colleague contacts, and from other key informants. These people were mostly in the United States and in the United Kingdom. Several short conferences on residential child care and child welfare provided useful contextual information to the investigation.

Interviews were semi-structured on an individual basis and documented in field diaries. The interviews and conferences were later written up in some detail in a separate document, used for analysis.

Piloting the Involvement of Young People in Staff Selection

A pilot project was initiated to explore directly the process of involving young people in and from care in staff selection. This was seen as qualitatively different from other situations in child welfare practice in which a sole client may have sat on a staff selection panel.

Five trials were undertaken. They included young people from the ages of 13 to 22 in selection panel groups of two and three, in the recruitment of care staff, youth workers, and an education worker. In addition, one trial was run with parents from a family support program participating in selecting a new family support worker. The five trials utilized situations that presented themselves in various workplaces within residential child care and in other welfare programs.

The research was thus undertaken by practice examples in real-life situations; the work, by its very nature, involved collaboration with the young people and, to some extent, with the job applicants; and the learning from each trial was logically applied to those following, in order to improve practice and iron out difficulties. Following this preparatory work, the first trial was undertaken. The subsequent trials formed a progressive spiral of action, observation, reflection, and planning further action.

Analysis

A process of inductive analysis (Patton, 1990) was adopted. The research began with specific observations and built progressively towards general patterns. Open-ended questions led to ideas not previously considered and to the pursuit of new paths of discovery as they emerged.

Analysis of the research data was undertaken using methods described by Krueger (1988) for the focus groups and Patton (1990) for the study tour. Analysis of the pilot project was undertaken using a reflective process as described by Kemmis and McTaggert (1988).

Chapter 4

Key Principles of Quality Care

The principles of quality residential care as identified have been grouped into the following categories: child-centered issues, staffing, organizational issues, and "the field."

CHILD-CENTERED ISSUES

A Child-Centered Model of Care

> Generally, the more child-centered and overtly caring the regime, the better the outcome for children, from the point of view of their education, personal growth, development and social conduct. (Bullock, Little, & Millham, 1993, cited in Support Force for Children's Residential Care, 1995b, p. 17)

The model for a residential child care program should be based, first of all, on an understanding of the developmental needs of children and young people and on an understanding of the particular and individual needs of abused and neglected children (Beedell & Clough, 1992). Planning for educational and special needs is a part of this. The aim should be to provide care which is as close as possible to that provided by families in their own homes and to provide the essential functions of "holding, nurturing and development of self" (Beedell & Clough, 1992, p. 2). The crucial role of the child's own family needs to be recognized. "The children's needs should dictate the standards, not the traditions of the service providers" (Kahan, personal communication, 1994).

[Haworth co-indexing entry note]: "Key Principles of Quality Care." Kiraly, Meredith. Co-published simultaneously in *Child & Youth Services* (The Haworth Press, Inc.) Vol. 23, No. 1/2, 2001, pp. 59-67; and: *Residential Child Care Staff Selection: Choose with Care* (Meredith Kiraly) The Haworth Press, Inc., 2001, pp. 59-67. Single or multiple copies of this article are available for a fee from The Haworth Document Delivery Service [1-800-HAWORTH 9:00 a.m. - 5:00 p.m. (EST). E-mail address: getinfo@haworthpressinc.com].

A Family and Community-Focused Approach to Children and Young People

Child welfare research testifies to the damaging effect of residential care practice that does not seek actively to maintain the family connections of children and young people (Millham, Bullock, Hosie, & Haak, 1986; Tresiliotis & Russell, 1984). This is particularly true in the light of research which shows that, contrary to the impressions of many workers, 9 out of 10 young people return home from residential care (Bullock, Little, & Millham, 1993), but that return is very stressful and frequently subject to breakdown. A family-focused approach is crucial to the well-being of children in care (Maluccio, Fein, & Olmstead, 1986).

Parents articulated repeatedly their needs:

- to be listened to;
- to feel welcome in the residential units;
- for an understanding and non-judgmental approach to their difficulties;
- for detailed information about their children;
- for effective and frequent communication;
- for respect, acknowledgement and co-operation;
- for assistance and support with parenting tasks;
- for a commitment to openness and honesty in their communications with staff.

The job thus needs to be seen as wider than the direct daily care of children. The development of job descriptions needs to reflect a family-focused approach, and staff need to be adequately trained and resourced if they are to work with families.

The social network of the child or young person is broader than the immediate family. It includes an awareness of extended family, the child's peer group–existing and potential–and children's links to their community. Staff need to be proactive in exploring with the child opportunities to build and maintain contacts with family, friends and people in the community.

A Recognition of the Critical Importance of Continuity of Care

The literature is very clear regarding the critical importance of continuity of care (Goldstein, Freud, & Solnit, 1973; Maluccio, Fein, &

Olmstead, 1986). Young people and parents bore vivid witness to this pain. Young people's comments included:

- Change is very hard for kids, and repeated change is very difficult.
- Okay, it's a real shit but I guess we accept it because at the end of the day we knew we were not a 100% real family, that was part of the deal.
- They should keep in touch and take an interest after they leave.

Similarly, a residential worker said, "Continuity is very important to the kids. Constant change is terrible for them. Good staff should be looked after for the sake of the children."

Both recruitment and selection strategies need to be oriented to the need to minimize staff turnover.

Effective Monitoring of Care

Effective case planning has long been recognized as essential to quality care. Considerable energy in recent years has gone into local attempts to ensure that case planning is timely, thorough, and professionally-based. Nevertheless, the process at times still lacks an empowering approach to children and their families. Parents called for limited numbers of participants in case-planning meetings, accurate and respectfully-written reports, and consideration in the way issues are raised, discussed and resolved.

A British system for monitoring the out-of-home care of children has recently been finalized after many years of research. This system, *Looking After Children* (Ward, 1995), addresses in detail both case-planning and the monitoring of care across the range of dimensions of the life of a child or young person from a participatory perspective. A system like this needs to be in place to ensure that care staff are guided adequately in terms of the specific tasks and expectations of the job and that families' needs are considered in the monitoring process.

Children's Rights and Involvement

> Yeah, I believe that everybody should have a say in who should look after them . . . I'll give VAYPIC a steer here! That is what VAYPIC is about . . . It is to give kids that are in care confidence in speaking out about who they want to look after them and what they

> think their needs are, like to be able to be heard, and choosing your own staff is being heard, you know? (Young person in focus group)

The issue of children's rights was raised repeatedly by participants in the focus groups and key informants during the study tour, in relation to how to improve the quality of residential child care.

The rights of children in care were frequently overlooked in the past (Kahan, 1979). Children's rights are being increasingly recognized as important to quality residential child care (Australian Association of Young People in Care, 1994; Canadian Youth in Care Network, 1994; Kiraly, 1994; Lindsay, personal communication, 1994; McCaughan, 1992; Victorian Association of Young People in Care, undated). Children's rights include the right to time, care and respect from staff, the right to be consulted about their care and planning for their present and future, the right to appropriate advocates when needed or wanted, and the right to be involved in the development of decisions and policy about the care offered (Australian Association of Young People in Care, 1984, p. 8).

A recognition of children's rights and the need for user-friendly complaints processes that will be acted upon quickly are crucial elements of the prevention of abuse in care (Platt, personal communication, 1994). Recent literature suggests that they may have a valuable role to play in child welfare staff selection (Berridge & Wenman, 1995; Lindsay, 1995).

STAFFING

Excellent Staff

The skills and personal qualities of the staff are the central features of quality care. Ensuring excellent staffing is a result of a range of good recruitment, selection, staff support, and management practices.

Appropriate Staffing Models

Effective staffing depends on staffing models that are viable and allow staff to do their best work without becoming overburdened by stress or fatigue. In particular, they need to have shifts that are not too long and sufficient support or team staff to share the load. The particular problems this presents for the family group home model need to be addressed. There is increasing recognition by agencies and funding bodies that family group home carers need more help in the form of support staff and more breaks from duty if they are to manage the care of increasingly challenging children and young people.

An Understanding of the Characteristics of a Skilled Child Care Worker

The question of the skills required by a residential child care worker needs to be addressed (Beker, personal communication, 1994; Stuck, personal communication, 1994). While certain key personal attributes are necessary, competent child care workers have a wide range of different personalities and personal styles (Peters & Getz, 1986). Therefore, the focus should be both on personal attributes and on specific and necessary skills.

Professional Development as a Life-Long Activity

There is now substantial recognition across the English-speaking world of the need for formal training for residential child care staff (e.g., Brasse, 1994; Madge, 1994; VanderVen, personal communication, 1994). Training needs to be provided both before and during employment to assist staff to deal constructively and creatively with the many challenges of residential child care. The capacity and willingness of staff to continue to utilize learning opportunities is required. It is also important that effective selection is not seen as a substitute for comprehensive training.

Care and Support of Staff

There is widespread concern among authorities in the child welfare field that residential child care staff are not adequately supported and supervised and that support for staff is frequently neglected, including supervision and appraisal, appropriate training, complaints procedures and grievance processes, financial resources, clear policy guidelines, and moral and practical support. Recruitment and selection is only part of the process of ensuring quality care. Unless staff are consistently supported, improvements in staff selection practices will be wasted.

ORGANIZATIONAL ISSUES

An Agency Culture of Continuous Improvement

Change is occurring in the child welfare field at a rapid rate, and practice needs to be based on the knowledge gained from child welfare research. Agencies need to be in touch with field developments and be willing and sufficiently resourced to implement these if quality care is to be achieved.

An Open, Effective, and Supportive Management Structure

Much evidence points to the clear link between organizational climate and management structures and the delivery of quality care (Cashmore, Dolby, McGregor, 1994; Clough, 1986; Forward, 1995). At its worst, a poor organizational structure can lead to abuse of children in care (Wyre, 1996). Staff performance is closely linked to the kind of environment in which they work (Murphy, 1994; Peters & Madle, 1991). An effective management structure includes good strategic planning and information systems (Brasse, personal communication, 1994), regular supervision and performance review systems (Beedel & Clough, 1992), and the involvement of outsiders to the organization in programs (Clough, 1986).

Clear and Accessible Procedures for Dealing with Allegations of Abuse

Even with the best system of staff selection, there may be cases of abuse in care. It is the view of experts in personnel selection that there is no fool-proof way of ensuring that a pedophile will not "slip through" the selection net (Fletcher, personal communication, 1994; Platt, personal communication, 1994). Clear policy guidelines need to be in place, together with the resources needed, for allegations of abuse in care to be dealt with quickly and effectively (Cavanagh, 1991).

Staff need to be advised of their responsibility under *Duty of Care* (a legal responsibility in Australia, the United States, and the United Kingdom) to whistle-blow if necessary and should be supported through this process. A policy should be in place to support the process (Support Force for Children's Residential Care, 1995a).

Clear Policy Guidelines and Standards

Staff need to have clear policy guidelines and codes of practice for a range of areas of day-to-day practice, including minimum standards expected. Policy needs to be developed collaboratively over time with staff, it should be documented, and it should be reviewed periodically. An Australian national standard, *Baseline Out-of-Home Care Standards* (Standing Committee of Community Services and Income Security Administrators, 1995) provides some broad-brush guidelines for developing standards in agencies.

THE FIELD

A Conscious Countering of the Poor Image of Residential Child Care

The international scene reflects local experience of the low status and poor image of residential child care. In the United Kingdom, a series of research and practice initiatives are underway to counter this poor image. The Support Force for Children's Residential Care, the National Children's Bureau, the Dartington Social Research Unit, and the Centre for Residential Child Care (Glasgow) are some of the major bodies behind this practice-based research. It is a widely-held view that quality care will never be fully achievable until the importance of the service, the need for adequate resourcing, and the quality of care that can be offered given the right conditions are recognized by professional organizations, funding bodies, and the general community. Residential care is a "positive choice" for some youth (Hendley, 1994; Wagner, 1987), and the huge demands of caring for the most challenging children in the child protection system need to be recognized (Berridge, 1992b, p. 236).

A Clear Sense of Purpose

> Residential care should not be regarded as the option of last resort when all else fails. It should have a clearly defined purpose and ethos offering specific support for specific needs. (Audit Commission, 1994, cited in Support Force for Children's Residential Care, 1995b)

Quality residential care is only possible when there is recognition in the child welfare field of its value in the range of out-of-home care options, and an understanding of when it is best used (Lane, 1983; Brasse, 1994; Clough, 1994). While supporting the retention of residential care for the most challenging placements, present directions in out-of-home care in Victoria are tending to reduce the use of residential child care as far as possible and to use it as the placement of last resort. In the United Kingdom (Clough, personal communication, 1994) and the United States (Magnuson, personal communication, 1994), there has been a tendency to revisit the move away from residential care and to seek to use residential care earlier in a child's out-of-home life. A more positive sense of purpose, whether in responding to the most challenging placements or in a more inclusive agenda, would assist in improving the quality of care locally.

Sufficient Financial Resources

This is a continuing issue in the residential child care field. The field continues to struggle to gain access to secure funding at a level sufficient to ensure quality care. Quality care costs money and cannot be provided when the over-riding motive is to save money. The current economic climate makes achievement of high standards in residential child care staffing and programming particularly difficult. In 1994, Murphy wrote:

> While the availability of adequate funding is an issue, underlying and contributing to this issue is the preparedness of agencies to operate inadequately funded programs. This practice is a sanction for funding bodies to withhold the provision of adequate levels of financial support to agencies for their residential programs. (p. 32)

The situation is the same now.

Professionalization

Many of the problems of residential child care are related to the engagement of untrained staff to take on one of the most skilled and challenging jobs in the human services field. The European experience suggests that the incidence of poor standards and abuse in care may be directly related to the failure to acknowledge residential child care as another of the child care professions alongside teaching and youth work.

Formal recognition of residential child care as a profession is a long way off in Australia and the English-speaking world. Nevertheless, child welfare professionals need to look and work towards a future when residential child care is professionalized. Thorough training, both as a pre-requisite to service as well as in-service, needs to be a goal.

There remains a place in the care of children and young people for the talented but unqualified residential child care worker who is open to continuous learning (Beedell & Clough, 1992). A future goal should be to offer all such workers viable opportunities to train to professional standards while in service (Kelly & Payne, personal communication, 1994).

Chapter 5

Principles of Good Staff Selection

GENERAL PRINCIPLES

The Assignment of Adequate Time to the Process

> . . . our experience would suggest that appointments are often made late, on occasion because appointments to fill vacancies are deferred to save money; and then with great urgency because the staff and children badly need the cover . . . a hurried and pressed context for appointments must be risky. (Beedell & Clough, 1992, p. 7)

Tom Peter's (1988) first rule for recruitment and interviewing is "spend time and lots of it" (p. 379). All the knowledge of good practice and technique will be of little value if the time and attention to the task is insufficient for the various tasks of staff selection to be carried out thoroughly. Participants in the focus groups also made this point. Two to three months is needed to undertake a thorough selection from the time the job is reviewed and advertised until the time the appointee commences work (Victorian Council of Social Service, 1993).

Validity

A model of staff selection must be as reliable and valid as possible. Reliability and validity are very difficult issues to measure in practice. Therefore, it is important to build upon the extensive research knowledge in personnel selection and to utilize processes with validity. In order to transfer knowledge effectively from personnel selection, the model must also embrace an understanding of the context of contemporary residential care.

[Haworth co-indexing entry note]: "Principles of Good Staff Selection." Kiraly, Meredith. Co-published simultaneously in *Child & Youth Services* (The Haworth Press, Inc.) Vol. 23, No. 1/2, 2001, pp. 69-82; and: *Residential Child Care Staff Selection: Choose with Care* (Meredith Kiraly) The Haworth Press, Inc., 2001, pp. 69-82. Single or multiple copies of this article are available for a fee from The Haworth Document Delivery Service [1-800-HAWORTH 9:00 a.m. - 5:00 p.m. (EST). E-mail address: getinfo@haworthpressinc.com].

An Understanding of the Job and Needed Skills

Before effective selection can occur, it is important to be clear about what the job of residential child care worker entails. Job analysis should be thorough and lead to an up-to-date job description and person specification. In order to write the "person specification," it is important to be clear about the skills and characteristics of a skilled residential child care worker. This research study led to the development of a profile of a skilled residential child care worker as one of its outcomes, described in Appendix D.

A Standard Involving Multiple Measures

Interviews and reference checks alone are not sufficient. A work test or other device that is closely related to the job requirements is needed Also, appropriate preparation and follow-up to the selection process is needed for best practice to occur. A standard for good staff selection thus needs to be set.

Ethics and Confidentiality

Methods of collecting, storing, and communication of information in the staff selection process need to reflect professional standards (Anderson & Shackleton, 1993, p. 25). The process of selection is two-way; the way applicants are treated also affects the image of the agency and thus its capacity to recruit the best staff (De Witte, 1989; Wendover, 1989).

The Involvement of Residential Care Staff and Clients

Focus group participants favor involving residential staff in the selection of new staff. This was seen as common-sense good practice, although it is not typical. A number of staff in the focus groups spoke of the capacity of residential staff to know by a process of "gut feeling" whether an applicant would be suitable for the job. Comments from care staff included:

- You get vibes from the person you are interviewing.
- You just know, don't you?
- You can feel it, can't you?

Client involvement in carer selection is now seen as a *right* by members of the advocacy groups of young people in care in different parts of the world. Staff in child welfare services are increasingly recognizing and supporting this claim (Berridge & Wenman, 1995). It is also seen as a practice that is likely to make a significant impact on the quality of selection decisions. Early pilots of this approach in the United Kingdom and Australia suggest that young people have a unique perspective to offer in evaluating the interpersonal skills of candidates in relation to young people (Lindsay & Rayner, 1993).

Equal Employment Opportunity (EEO)

Considerable restrictions are placed upon the process of staff selection by EEO guidelines. These ensure that only job-relevant criteria are taken into consideration in the selection decision, thus increasing the accuracy of decision-making. Where the specific needs of children in care conflict with formal EEO requirements, there is provision in Australia and many other countries to seek an EEO exemption.

The Need for Training in Staff Selection

The body of expertise about effective interviewing and other staff selection practices has not translated into better practice in the community (Anderson & Shackleton, 1993). If staff selection practice is to be improved, training is necessary. Various research studies bear witness to the difficulty of designing training packages that are effective in improving staff selection practice. Training courses should be based upon available research knowledge, be of reasonable duration, for example, 1-2 days, and be workshop-based, that is, allowing for skill practice. The unique aspects of residential child care also need to be addressed.

Varied workplaces, philosophies of care, and positions require different job descriptions and possibly different staff selection techniques.

TECHNICAL PRINCIPLES

Appropriate Self-Assessment

Self-assessment and self-selection, under the right conditions, empower the applicant and enhances the chances of obtaining the best applicant for the job. It needs to be done early in the process, outside of the interview, and on the basis of adequate information about the position (Hesketh, personal communication, 1994; Wanous, 1982). A Realistic Job Preview (RJP) assists with the process of self-assessment and helps to set reasonable expectations of the job (Gardner, Foo, & Hesketh, 1995; Hesketh, 1994).

Improvements to the Selection Interview and the Reference Check

Since the selection interview and the reference check are likely to remain the most widely-used selection tools, it makes sense to direct energy towards their improvement based upon research knowledge. Interview processes have been slow to improve by comparison with other selection methods. Improvements can be made at relatively little cost compared with the development of other assessment tools (Robertson & Makin, 1993).

Use Work Tests and De-Emphasize Psychological Testing

Including appropriate work tests is the best way to improve the selection process for residential child care workers. Doing so is more effective than adding psychological tests to the mix. Numerous studies in the United States over the last twenty years attempted to establish the utility of existing or customized psychological tests for determining the profile of a competent residential child care worker. None of these studies have achieved this to an adequate level of validity. British child welfare practitioners have similarly concluded that a suitable test for this field does not yet exist (Anderson, 1994; United Kingdom Deparment of Health, 1992).

An Effective Decision-Making Model

> Interviewers are the major source of error, being prone to a variety of dysfunctions in their information-processing strategies. (Anderson & Shackleton, 1993, p. 68)

While staff selection techniques and processes can be improved and multiple processes put in place, none of these processes will in themselves lead to accurate decision-making. The final decision needs to be made upon the weight of information collected in a structured way and with awareness of the various causes of decision-making bias.

A Thorough Strategy for Deterring Abusers

There is increasing awareness about the risk that pedophiles and other abusive individuals pose to children and young people in residential care. There is also concern that some pedophiles will be able to succeed in passing all the best selection strategies and screening devices. Thus, some organizations have turned to developing systematic ways to deter such people from continuing to seek employment in residential care (Waldron, personal communication, 1994, Support Force for Children's Residential Care, 1995b). Methods of deterring unsuitable persons are dealt with elsewhere in this publication.

THE DECISION-MAKING PROCESS

The process of decision-making is as much of a problem in effective staff selection as are the methods of selection utilized (Anderson, 1994). Hakel (1989) says, "Interrater agreement is *the* key issue" (p. 291). Anderson (personal communication, 1994) says, in regard to how decisions are made by interview panels, "The main problem is in the information-processing and decision-making area." Decision-making error may be reduced by a number of general strategies as well as by some which are specific to the decision-making phase of staff selection. General strategies include:

- Allowing adequate time for this, the most important phase of the selection process (Staley, Ranck, Perreault, & Neugebauer, 1986).
- Training selection panels in the common areas of bias in selection (Anderson & Shackleton, 1993).
- The use of multiple methods of assessment rather than the interview and reference check alone to add incremental validity (Kahan; personal communication, 1994; Kelly & Payne, personal communication, 1994).
- Basing interviews upon detailed job analysis and a clear job description and person specification using a structured interviewing format (Pursell, Campion, & Gaylord, 1980).
- Selecting the selection panel according to EEO principles and relevant experience in both the field and in staff selection.
- Using a simple and clear method of documentation of selection decisions for future reference and in case of legal or other challenge of the decision.

Specific strategies to reduce decision-making error include:

- Throughout the decision-making phase, intentional questioning of prejudices and prevailing myths about the sort of person who makes a good carer (Commissioner for Equal Opportunity, 1978; VanderVen, personal communication, 1994).
- Using arithmetic forms of evaluation, such as rating scales, for all selection tests (Anderson & Shackleton, 1993). The simplest forms of ratings are probably as effective as more complicated ones (Giffin, 1989; Janz, 1982).
- Rating applicants on performance rating scales prior to discussing their performance in a selection panel is very important if bias is to be avoided (Fletcher, personal communication, 1994); otherwise the negative dynamics of the group will interfere (Anderson, 1994). The selection panel has the potential to use group process to confirm the prejudices of one or more of its members.
- Selection panels should be trained in the common errors in interviewer ratings and in the use of rating scales themselves (Anderson & Shackleton, 1993).
- Applicants should not be discussed prior to interview (Anderson, 1994).
- Dipboye (1989) says that post-interview impressions tend to conform to pre-interview impressions, and that "the interview seems most likely to contribute to the prediction of a criterion to the extent that the information gathered during this phase is kept independent of information gathered in the first phase and considered on its own merit" (p. 49). This suggests that there may be some merit in the selection panel not previewing applications. However, Anderson (1994), Fletcher (personal communication, 1994), and Harris (personal communication, 1994) feel that this is an impracticable idea. At the least, it would seem appropriate for the selection panel to discuss the potential for previewing the application forms to lead to bias and to consciously guard against this.
- Longer interviews seem to lead to a more considered judgment than shorter ones (Tullar, Mullins, & Caldwell, 1979).
- The number of interviews done in one day should be limited to about four, in order to reduce bias generated from fatigue, boredom, and inattentiveness (Maurer & Fay, 1988).
- The use of follow-up questioning, or another interview, to follow-up concerns or misgivings is to be encouraged (Staley, Ranck, Perreault, & Neugebauer, 1986).

EQUAL EMPLOYMENT OPPORTUNITY (EEO)

EEO issues appear repeatedly in the personnel selection literature. In the United Kingdom and United States it has been a large political issue in personnel selection over many years, with most of the concern being related to issues of sex and race. In Australia, to date most issues that have come to the attention of the Anti-discrimination Tribunal in Victoria have been related to issues of gender (Commissioner for Equal Opportunity, 1992).

Clear guidelines outline requirements of employers with regard to EEO. However, residential child care is exempt, by statute, from some EEO requirements. For example, in Melbourne, at Anglicare Victoria, the agency operates two gender-specific residential units for abused young women under EEO exemptions, that is, all staff must be female.

The specific findings of this study are specific and numerous:

- In general, the requirement to adhere to EEO legislation has the benefit of ensuring that only job-relevant criteria are taken into consideration in the selection decision, thus improving the decision-making outcome (Beedell & Clough, 1992; VCOSS, 1993).
- Where a particular job is regarded as stereotypically female, there is considerable evidence of prejudice against male applicants in employment decisions (Campion & Arvey, 1989). This may apply to residential care in a number of settings; therefore, it is important to watch for bias against male applicants. Further, there is a risk of discriminating against males in an attempt to avoid recruiting a pedophile (Pringle, 1993).
- It is important to encourage diversity in staff in terms of ethnicity (Waldron, 1994) and to consciously question prevailing myths about stereotypes of good workers (Commissioner for Equal Opportunity, 1978). It is also important to provide for a balance of caring male and female role models for children in care (Beedell & Clough, 1992) to allow for appropriate protection of privacy and to respond sensitively to children's anxieties as a result of abuse. This can be done by implementing EEO principles and applying for legal exemptions where needed.
- Some tensions may at times apparently exist between EEO provisions as written and best practice. For example, it may be seen as beneficial to have only female staff in an emergency residential unit for sexually-abused young women or, conversely, it may be desirable to have dedicated male and female staff in a residential

unit where it is seen as important to have effective role-modelling by staff of both genders. As mentioned above, legal exemptions from EEO requirements may be available to cover these situations in a number of countries.

- In Australia, sex and marital status discrimination is sometimes permitted under Section 35 of the *Sex Discrimination Act* (Australia, 1984). It may thus be possible to discriminate on the basis of marital status should an agency wish to insist on this as a role model. Accommodation provided by a religious body, charitable, or non-profit body may be exempt at times under Section 23 of the same act (Commissioner for Equal Opportunity, 1992). In the accommodation field, there is also provision under Section 30 of the *Equal Opportunity Act* (Victoria, 1995) such that the accommodation may not be used for a child if its design or location is deemed unsuitable. These latter provisions may have implications for the birth children of family group home staff.
- Staff should be recruited on the presumption that as far as possible and appropriate, all tasks should be shared equally between male and female staff, except where the privacy of children dictate otherwise (Beedell & Clough, 1992).
- A detailed job analysis leading to a clear job description and person specification is an EEO requirement in the United States (Pearn & Kandola, 1988) and is good practice anywhere. It is likely to minimize discrimination caused by considering information that is not job-relevant (Dessler, 1988).
- The selection panel should be designed being mindful of the need to minimize discrimination. Therefore, there should be at least one male and one female and preferably a person from a non-English-speaking background (Campion & Arvey, 1989; United Kingdom Department of Health, 1992).
- It is important to work from a standardized interview schedule where the same questions are asked of all applicants; however, flexibility should also be allowed in order to follow-up responses. Rigid interview processes lead to using reduced information to make a decision (Thomas, personal communication, 1994).
- Information needed to determine job suitability and reasonable availability to work, even some personal information, can be requested by the use of appropriate wording of questions that do not discriminate (Murray, 1986; Pecora & Austin, 1987). Similarly, questions regarding relevant life experiences may be asked if

phrased carefully to make their job-relevance clear (Commissioner for Equal Opportunity, 1986).

- Decisions regarding rejection of a person on the basis of a criminal records check should take into consideration the benefit of having on staff individuals who may have had life difficulties in their adolescence or young adulthood, including minor convictions irrelevant to the job, providing that there is evidence that the issues which led to their offending are resolved.

JOB ANALYSIS

Job analysis is defined as "the process of examining a job in order to identify its component parts" (Anderson & Shackleton, 1993, p. 17). In the personnel selection literature it is a crucial component of an effective staff selection strategy (Equal Employment Opportunity Commission, 1978; Pfau, 1990). Lack of clarity about the objectives of the establishment and the task are common reasons for wasting staff (O'Brien, 1994). Good practice in this area is often overlooked.

The findings of this study and the associated recommended practices are:

- Effective job analysis improves the accuracy of interview decisions (Wiesner & Cronshaw, 1988), the validity of personnel selection processes (Harris, 1989), and the reduction of bias against minority groups (Pursell, Campion, & Gaylord, 1980).
- The staff selection process should start from a detailed job analysis with an intermediate level of specificity, taking a strategic or future-oriented approach, that is, looking at future changes to the job (Hesketh, 1994; Schneider & Konz, 1989). This is particularly relevant to residential child care where the job varies from agency to agency and change is occurring at a rapid pace. For example, in some agencies where staff are expected to take a stronger role in working with parents of children in care, the job description will need to be quite different.
- The method needs to be efficient in terms of time and cost. Options include a semi-structured group staff interview, a questionnaire to staff, or a combination of both (Pearn & Kandola, 1988). Group interviews, including residential care staff of more than one agency, would allow cross-fertilization of ideas about the nature of the job and future possibilities.

- The job analysis should lead to a clear job description written to a standardized *pro forma* that is clear, specific, and brief and indicates the scope of the job (Dessler, 1988).
- In the residential child care field, it is important to be clear about the nature of the task, including its strong affective/emotional content, and the potential of this to affect staff (Clough, 1994).
- As important as an outcome of the job analysis is the development of a clear and detailed person specification that converts the duties and responsibilities of the job description into a set of selection criteria. This becomes the standard against which applicants' qualifications and experience will be assessed (Dessler, 1988). The United Kingdom Department of Health (1992) advocates the use of person specifications that clearly specify essential and desirable attributes. This report suggests that these two categories are frequently confused, resulting in wrong judgments about suitability.

It is important to be clear about the skills and attributes that are needed in a residential child care worker. There is a tendency to see little difference between a good carer and a "nice person" (Stuck, personal communication, 1994). Skills and attributes required will vary according to different program philosophies. Young people in care may be able to assist with identifying relevant skills and characteristics. Cognitive skills need to be appreciated as part of the profile (VanderVen, personal communication, 1994).

The following are the priorities identified by children in care and their parents regarding the job of the residential child care worker:

- to provide stability, consistency, and some continuity over time in children's lives;
- to provide care, friendship, and support;
- to provide guidance and encouragement in children's lives and activities;
- to listen and discuss things;
- to be there when you need them–everything;
- to treat children as individuals;
- to provide a feeling of family as much as possible;
- to be fun;
- to keep parents involved as much as possible but not to push families together;

- to communicate in detail with parents as much as possible about their children and to co-operate with them when possible; and
- to understand parents' problems and circumstances and to try to support them as much as possible.

Summary

A detailed job analysis is an essential part of an effective recruitment and selection strategy in residential child care. It should look to both the existing job and to future developments and be effective in terms of time and cost. Client input is important in the process of a job analysis for residential child care. Based on the job analysis, a clear job description and person specification needs to be developed.

THE QUESTION OF PSYCHOLOGICAL TESTING

Psychological testing as a personnel selection method is not commonly used in Australia, with the exception of some use in executive selection in private enterprise (Parkes, 1985; Saul, 1980). Psychological testing did, however, emerge frequently in the literature reviews from the United States and has been tested there in residential child care staff selection. In addition, one of the more controversial recommendations of the United Kingdom Warner Inquiry was that personality tests be used to screen applicants for senior positions in residential child care and that efforts be made to develop appropriate tests to screen for the potential to sexually abuse children (United Kingdom Department of Health, 1992). This has led to a great increase in the industry of psychological testing by consulting companies in relation to residential child care staff selection in the United Kingdom (Anderson, 1994).

Because of this strong international interest and activity in psychological testing for residential child care staff selection, this needs more detailed consideration.

Review of Psychological Tests Which Have Been Used in Residential Child Care Staff Selection

The following list includes tests that have been known to have been used in residential child care staff selection since 1980.

Child Abuse Potential Inventory, 2nd Edition, Joel S. Milner Psytec Inc., De Kalb, Illinois, United States (Milner, 1986). This test was constructed, trialed, and recommended by Milner and Wimberley (1979; 1980). Further studies suggest it is unsuitable for the screening of residential child care workers (Haddock & McQueen, 1983; Hart, 1989; Melton, 1989).

SRI Child Care Perceiver, Selection Research Inc., Lincoln, Nebraska, United States (Selection Research Inc., 1982). This is a structured interview with clear scoring criteria. Ross and Hoeltke (1985; 1987) did a large study (over 100 subjects) of the selection of residential child care workers in the United States. The results claimed for the Perceiver seemed impressive; there were significant correlations with self-ratings, supervisors' ratings, child resident ratings, and institutional climate. A study for EEO Acceptability revealed that the Perceiver seemed to be free of bias for age, race and gender.

An Australian trial of the Child Care Perceiver, in 1991, suggested that it might need substantial adaptation for Australian use. The Child Care Perceiver is still apparently in current, although apparently infrequent use, in the United States (Baker, personal communication, 1996; Showalter, personal communication, 1990). Reasons for its apparent lack of use in the United States given published results are unclear, although the significant costs of purchase and training may be a deterrent.

California Personality Inventory (Megargee 1972). Mufson (1986) used the California Psychological Inventory (CPI) to determine whether a high-functioning group of residential child care workers would display different characteristics from a low-functioning group. Mufson's total sample was 45; the final sample was 28. No further research on the use of the CPI in residential child care has been found.

Sixteen Personality Factor Questionnaire (16PF) (Cattel, Eber and Tatsuoka, 1980). Wasmund and Tate (1988) explored the discriminant properties of the 16PF to discern the personality characteristics of high-functioning versus low-functioning residential child care workers. Five of the 16PF factors were found to differentiate most from least effective child care workers. However, the overall constellation of personality factors only predicted high performance correctly 70% of the time. This may relate in part to the unreliability of the supervisors' ratings used as the criterion variable. Walsh (cited in Buros, 1978) concluded that the 16PF is a failure and impossible to recommend for any use from the most basic research to the most programatically-oriented applications.

Personnel Selection Inventory (London House, 1980). The Personnel Selection Inventory is a tool for predicting behaviors of residential child care workers. Jones, Joy and Martin (1990) recommend that the PSI be used with other credible selection devices such as interviews, reference checks, and effective monitoring programs. The validation studies of the PSI (Jones and Joy, 1987; Jones, Joy, & Martin, 1980) are encouraging but small, and criterion variables suffer from validity problems themselves, because the criterion measures were other tests that had not been validated as able to predict skill in residential child care.

Occupational Personality Questionnaire (OPQ) (Saville and Holdsworth, 1984). This tool is in current use in the United Kingdom (Anderson, 1994; Thomas, personal communication, 1994) and likely to be used increasingly as a result of recommendations in the Warner Report (United Kingdom Department of Health, 1992). No validation studies on residential child care workers have been done. Some in the United Kingdom are concerned about the vigorous marketing of this test, which exploits a tendency for unwarranted faith in test results. Also, the test is transparent and is likely to be easy to fake. The company that produces this test has a good reputation but no specific expertise in selecting people for human services positions.

General Considerations in Psychological Testing

Despite our best wishes, there is no test in existence will screen successfully for the potential for paedophilia or child sexual abuse (United Kingdom Department of Health, 1992; Fletcher, personal communication, 1994).

More hopefully, there is well-substantiated evidence of the validity of intelligence testing in predicting job performance (Barrett & Depinet, 1991; Hunter, 1986). In many situations, it would appear to out perform all other measures of job performance. While it has been argued that different jobs may require more or less general intelligence and thus that this finding may relate more to some jobs than others, Barrett and Depinet (1991) and Robertson and Makin (1993) say this finding is equally relevant to all work situations. VanderVen (personal communication, 1994) and Youdan (personal communication, 1994) are now arguing that the cognitive cluster of skills and the ability to learn is critical to good performance as a residential child care worker. While there may be insufficient reason to utilize intelligence testing in selecting residential care workers, cognitive skills should be assessed by asking relevant problem-solving questions in interviews, and they should be verified by reference checking.

A third area, personality testing, has been criticized by Barrick and Mount (1991) as a limited tool for predicting job performance. Even so, recent meta-analytical research has found that 3 of 5 "Big Personality Factors" do correlate with job performance. In particular, the personality construct of Conscientiousness (a strong sense of purpose, obligation, and persistence) shows a consistent relationship with all job performance criteria for all occupational groups. Openness to Experience is also correlated with cognitive ability or intelligence and, with Extraversion, correlates with training proficiency. Two of these qualities link clearly to qualities identified as important for care workers: Conscientiousness is close to Appropriate Motivation and Commitment, and Openness to Experience shares characteristics with Conceptual Thinker. Intelligence, Conscientiousness, and Openness to Experience are qualities that should be sought in selecting residential child care workers.

SECTION B. CHOOSE WITH CARE: A RECRUITMENT GUIDE FOR ORGANIZATIONS WORKING WITH CHILDREN

Choose with Care: A Recruitment Guide for Organizations Working with Children

FOREWORD

I commend this book to all those employing people to work with children, whether for payment or otherwise. I recently had reason to contact the coordinator of a well established children's association to inquire what procedures were in place for checking out group leaders. The response was "None." It became clear that the State co-ordinator did not think that such precautions were either possible or necessary and that there was no child protection policy in place. Although one of his leaders had been reported (on several occasions) to child protection authorities for serious offences, the alleged offender was still working with boys at his local group. Pedophiles are constantly looking for sloppy organizations and careless parents; they justify their own criminal behavior by claiming that the responsible adults behaved irresponsibly, "leaving the kids with anybody." Apart from the

[Haworth co-indexing entry note]: "Choose with Care: A Recruitment Guide for Organizations Working with Children." Kiraly, Meredith. Co-published simultaneously in *Child & Youth Services* (The Haworth Press, Inc.) Vol. 23, No. 1/2, 2001, pp. 83-124; and: *Residential Child Care Staff Selection: Choose with Care* (Meredith Kiraly) The Haworth Press, Inc., 2001, pp. 83-124. Single or multiple copies of this article are available for a fee from The Haworth Document Delivery Service [1-800-HAWORTH 9:00 a.m. - 5:00 p.m. (EST). E-mail address: getinfo@haworthpressinc.com].

risks to children, organizations that fail to take basic precautions to protect their charges are at high risk of being sued for negligence should anyone in their organization, paid or volunteer, commit offences against juveniles. Increasingly, former victims are turning to the civil courts for compensation. Even parents employing child-minders should check out new employees with previous employers and their children. They should also ask children to express their gut feelings. Particular care must be taken when recruiting volunteers for camps for disadvantaged and disabled children and Sunday Schools. International studies have shown that children with disabilities are up to 700% more likely than non-disabled children to be victimized by child sex offenders. The greatest risk is from caregivers.

ECPAT and MacKillop Family Services are to be commended for producing this (long overdue) book. I hope that it is well used.

Freda Briggs
Professor of Child Development,
University of South Australia

I am extremely pleased to recommend this guide for the recruitment of personnel to work with children. It is the responsibility of all organizations working with children to ensure they are cared for and protected. Selection of staff is fundamental. This contribution will assist us all to do better and ensure children in our care are kept safe. I warmly recommend this guide.

Wendy Rose
National Director,
Save the Children Australia

The responsibility of any organization working with children to ensure a safe environment is a heavy one. Every single child is a precious human being, born free and possessed of an inherent dignity and worth that deserves protection and demands warm respect. Sadly, many millions of such precious children in our world are exposed to circumstances that render them vulnerable to exploitation and abuse. A civilization that cares will have many agencies committed to the protection and well-being of children at risk, but the discharge of that trust requires the skilled recruitment of workers, including volunteers, who understand what it means to share that trust and to respect the integrity of the child. I warmly recommend this Guide as a valuable contribution to that end and congratulate ECPAT and MacKillop on its content.

Sir Ronald Wilson, AC KBE CMG QC
President of the Australian Council for Overseas Aid

In the past, police regularly investigated child sexual assaults that may have been prevented if more thorough or conscientious screening processes had been applied during the recruitment of personnel. However, organizations with a duty of care for children are slowly realizing that duty by minimizing the potential for child molesters to be employed in their organizations. This manual is a positive step forward in the attempt to minimize the access of child molesters to children.

Detective Senior Sergeant Chris O'Connor
Head of Victoria (Australia) Police Child Exploitation Squad

ACKNOWLEDGEMENTS

The inspiration for this project came from Bernadette McMenamin, National Director, ECPAT Australia. ECPAT Australia has worked with organizations to raise awareness on this issue since 1994 and has run numerous workshops on preventing the employment of abusers.

Paul Linossier, CEO of MacKillop Family Services, provided strong support for the proposal and donated staff time for the writing of the project.

We acknowledge the funding that was provided for some of the initial research upon which this booklet draws. These funding sources were Kildonan Child and Family Services, the Creswick Foundation for Family Relations and Child Development, the Stegley Foundation, the Viertel Foundation, and the Felton Bequest.

Some of the ideas in this handbook were first written for *Recruiting and Selecting Residential Child Care Workers* (Kildonan Child and Family Services, 1999) and are drawn upon with permission.

The model of recruitment, selection and support is copyrighted by Goding Human Resources and is reproduced here with permission.

We also acknowledge and thank authorities in the United Kingdom and United States who provided consultations to support the development of a model of best practice in recruitment and selection. These people are:

In the UK: Mr. David Lane; Professor David Berridge; Dr. Mike Lindsay; Ms. Denise Platt; Ms. Susan Thomas; Professor Clive Fletcher; Dr. Neil Anderson; and Dr. Phil Youdan.

In North America: Mr. John Meston and Professor Burt Galaway (Canada); Professor Michael Harris; Ms. Ginnie Waldron; Dr. Tom Janz; Professor Jerry Beker; and Mr. Douglas Magnuson (USA).

ECPAT AUSTRALIA (CHILD WISE)

ECPAT Australia (End Child Prostitution, Pornography and Trafficking) is part of a global network of organizations working together for the elimination of the commercial sexual exploitation of children. ECPAT has bases in 48 countries. Since its inception on 1993, ECPAT Australia has focused on child sex tourism, child prostitution, child pornography, and sex trafficking of children. ECPAT Australia's work included community education and information provision, conducting national and international training programs, law reform and police development, promoting child-friendly tourism, and encouraging responsible provision and use of the internet. ECPAT Australia is a national campaign based in Melbourne. Its organizational base is Save the Children, World Vision, and Australian Volunteers International. Advisers to ECPAT include sector representatives from the judiciary, police, tourism, psychiatry, and human rights. ECPAT is in the process of a name change to Child Wise. It is available on the web at [www.ecpat.org]. It is available by e-mail at <ecpat@ecpat.org>, and by mail at ECPAT (Child Wise) Australia, P.O. Box 451, South Melbourne, Victoria, Australia 3205. The phone number is 61-3-9645-8911.

MACKILLOP FAMILY SERVICES

MacKillop Family Services is a child, youth, and family welfare agency operating in Victoria, Australia, and continues the work of the seven founding agencies formerly operated by the Mercy Sisters, the Christian Brothers and the Sisters of St. Joseph. MacKillop provides family support services to children and young people and their families, disability services, residential and home-based care for children and young people in need of protection, and education services. The organization's vision includes working with those who are most marginalized and at risk and a commitment to quality, innovation and advocacy. It is available on the web at [www.mackillop.org.au], by e-mail at <paul.linossier@mackillop.org.au>, by mail at MacKillop Family Services, 237 Cecil Street, South Melbourne, Victoria, Australia 3205, and by phone at 61-3-9699-9177.

ABOUT THE AUTHOR

Meredith Kiraly is a psychologist with twenty-five years experience in child and family programs in health, education, and welfare. In the last fifteen years she has been working in child, youth and family welfare services, particularly in residential care. She wrote this book while a program manager with MacKillop Family Services.

In the 1990s, she undertook a major research project on caregiver recruitment and selection. A Creswick Foundation Travelling Fellowship allowed her to visit the USA, the UK, Denmark, and Canada in 1994 to collect ideas from international authorities in both personnel selection and child/youth welfare. She has written *Recruiting and Selecting Residential Care Workers* (Kildonan Child and Family Services, 1999); *The Problem of the Paedophile: Guidelines for Recruiting Staff for Positions in Child and Youth Care,* a 1995 article for *Children Australia;* and other journal articles on youth welfare that have been published in Australia and the UK. She has also trained staff in recruitment and selection and given many conference papers on staff recruitment and other topics. She completed a Master of Behavioral Science on staff recruitment. She is currently doing project work for community services organizations, government, and tertiary institutions. Her e-mail address is <kiraly@melbpc.org.au>.

GLOSSARY

"A child" means every human being below the age of eighteen years unless, in the law applicable to the child, majority is attained earlier.

"Child sexual abuse" means any exploitation of a child, whether consensual or not, for the sexual gratification of a parent or person in whose care a child is and includes, but is not necessarily restricted to: sexual molestation, sexual assault, and the exploitation of the child for purposes of pornography or prostitution (Manitoba Community Services

1988, p. 14). It is recognized that the age for consensual sexual activity varies from country to country.

"A pedophile" is a significantly older individual who prefers to have sex with individuals legally considered children. "A child molester" is an individual who sexually molests children. These two things may be one and the same, or may not.

"Grooming" is the process of developing a trusting and affectionate relationship with a child, possibly over months, with the end goal of sexual abuse. The grooming process may include outings, activities, establishing rapport with the child's parents, and gradually introducing physical play and affectionate touch into the relationship, prior to actual sexual activity.

Situational Interview: A structured interview based upon questions that ask for responses to scenarios or hypothetical situations.

Behavioral Interview: A selection interview based upon asking the applicant for examples of job-relevant real life experiences and behavior from the applicant's past.

Realistic Job Preview (RJP): A process that provides a detailed picture of the job in question and stresses both the positive and negative aspects of the job and has been found to improve job satisfaction.

NGO: Non-Government Organization [in this context] delivering human services and/or aid programs.

INTRODUCTION

This handbook is written for non-government organizations that deliver development, aid, and child welfare programs both within Australia and internationally. It arises out of the ever increasing awareness that along with opportunities to make a difference to the lives of disadvantaged people comes the potential for child abuse–and that this has become a reality over time on too many occasions. Collectively, Australian society carries the weight of abuse of children of many backgrounds, including the Stolen Generation, within church and state institutions, within our schools, and through overseas aid projects. Through the work of ECPAT and other organizations we are now aware that this is a global problem and that abusers travel and network internationally in their search for avenues to vulnerable children and young people. Both staff and volunteers are implicated.

The acknowledgement of the extent of the problem of child sexual abuse is not intended to diminish the tremendous work of those individuals, paid and unpaid, who have given generously and professionally to further the well-being of disadvantaged people in many different ways. Rather, it is the beginning of an attempt to ensure that all, rather than most, who are given the privilege of working in human services use it to good ends.

Child Sexual Abuse

Child sexual abuse is a crime like no other. It targets the most vulnerable children and young people in the community. Children are dependent upon adults for love, security, food, clothing, shelter, and material goods. All of these basic needs lead to opportunities to give security and care–or for abuse. Affection, food, shelter, clothing, and money can be offered as gifts to entice or as rewards for sexual favors. Intoxicating and addictive substances can be introduced to reinforce the adult's power over the child by making them even more needy and dependent. Threats of violence, disclosure, or reprisal against family can be used to ensure compliance.

Further confusing the child, the long process of grooming in which care, affection, activities, and shared interests are slowly mixed with boundary-crossing touching and physical affection ensures that the child may be genuinely fond of the abuser and wish to please him or her. The child has sexual feelings that can be awakened to early adult-like expression, binding them in a sexually aroused state to their abuser, of whom they may have become fond, and on whom they are now dependent emotionally and materially. As awareness dawns on the child that there is something wrong with this form of sexual expression, the abuser uses–through blackmail–the child's ensuing guilt to further silence him or her. Given this process, it is not surprising to find that those children who have been abused and disclose their abuse are in the minority.

Human Services Agencies as a Target for Abusers

Agencies that work with disadvantaged children and families thus provide a plentiful source of children for the abuser to prey upon. Children can be targeted directly or through mentoring, support, and friendship with their parents or caregivers. This indirect route involves establishing trust with the child's parents or caretakers and ensures that the abuser's slowly increasing interest in the child will be supported and encouraged by those responsible for the child's care. The preferential child abuser may be practiced at the duplicity required to enter a community service organization and present as the very sensitive, caring, giving individual the organization is looking for. Abusers may be qualified or unqualified, have training in social welfare, trade skills, or no professional skills. Police statistics have enabled a profile to be developed of offenders with repeat convictions. However, it is variously estimated that between 1% and 5% of people who engage in acts of child molestation have a criminal record (Community Services Commission, 1996; Moriarty, 1990). There is no reliable profile of the overwhelming majority of unconvicted abusers (Staley, Ranck, Perreault, & Neugebauer, 1986).

Having painted this distressing picture, the aim of this handbook is to take a sensible rather than paranoid approach to the problem and not to assume that every applicant for human services work is likely to have ulterior motives. However, a real opportunity for the person with abusive intentions lies in an organization that has vague concepts of the person sought for a job, together with minimal selection procedures, followed up by management that is unaware of the opportunities it may afford for abuse within its program. Our aim then is to create an aware culture that will ensure the safety of children better than in the past and to do this within the limited resources which this sector has at its disposal.

Preferential and Situational Abusers

A preferential child abuser has a definite sexual preference for children. They have sex with children not because of some situational stress or insecurity but because they are sexually attracted to and prefer children. They have the potential to molest large numbers of victims (Lanning, 1986). This type is also called a pedophile.

A situational child abuser does not have a true sexual preference for children but engages in sex with children for varied and sometimes complex reasons. They may have fewer numbers of individual child victims, ranging from a single act to a long-term pattern of behavior. It is possible that this group is larger in number and increasing faster than the preferential child molester.

Pedophiles are responsible for the most publicized and scandalous examples of child abuse that come to light. However, it is likely that the second group is of even greater concern. More disturbingly, this second group may include a number of people who are distinguished from others in the community only by the fact of their going "over the line" of acceptable behavior, whether once or repeated. This can happen because of stress, provocation, poor supervision, or encouragement by others, whether child or adult.

In terms of prevention, the emphasis in management of the first group needs to be on deterring them from entering the field through the use of good selection procedures and ample information about the culture of the employing organization and then to have effective management in place in the unfortunate event that an abuser "slips through the net." With the second group, in addition to effective selection procedures that may eliminate clearly inappropriate applicants, the emphasis is on providing a climate where they are unlikely to offend or at worst will be apprehended straight away. This includes solid staff support, supervision, training, modelling of professional boundaries, clear policy, effective management, and user-friendly client complaints procedures.

Male and Female Offending

As far as we know, child sexual abuse is predominantly a male crime, with estimates ranging from 90% to 97% of perpetrators being male (Community Services Commission, 1996; McMenamin, 1996). We do not know very much about female child sexual abuse at the present time. Some authorities believe that it is more widespread than is yet widely recognized because "Women are primary caretakers in our society and can dress, bathe, change, examine and touch children with little suspicion" (Lanning, 1986, p. 10).

Recent cases in day child care have involved females, and there are many cases in which a female actively participates with a male accomplice.

Nevertheless, because at this time we believe this to be overwhelmingly a male crime, we use the pronoun "he" and "him" for the abuser in this handbook. We recognize that female child sexual abuse does occur. We also recognize that the vast majority of men in human services work are honorable and professional and carry in this era a heavy burden of suspicion because of the wrongs of others. We affirm their work and their essential role in modelling good, non-abusing care that disadvantaged children so sorely need.

THE AWARE CULTURE

The idea of an aware culture was developed in the United Kingdom by Ray Wyre (1996), a world authority on sexual offenders. An aware culture involves linking all aspects of the environment to ensure that the program is protective, enriches the lives of its children and families, and is clear about the boundaries between the personal and professional lives of staff. The following dimensions are important.

Relationship Between Staff and Children

Clear boundaries between roles. An awareness of the child's need for privacy in their bedroom and the bathroom. The sharing of outings with children among staff. One-to-one work between staff members and children to be done only by agreement and to be carefully monitored and supervised. Exclusiveness and secrecy challenged. No erotic or pornographic materials on premises. Confidentiality of documents relating to children's pasts and development. Open discussion among staff of appropriate and inappropriate behaviors in meetings and training sessions. Sensitivity to normal and inappropriate sexual expression in children and young people.

The Organization

An organization open to outside influence and accountability. Whistle-blowing policy acted upon appropriately. An environment that mitigates against influence, manipulation and secrecy, and confronts difficult issues. An appropriate physical environment that reduces the capacity to hide. Adequate communications systems, procedures, grievance and disciplinary processes that are enacted as needed. Proactive leadership and management. An awareness of the potential for female staff to abuse as well as males.

Staffing

Adequate staffing, staff supervision and training. Careful staff and volunteer selection procedures. Accountability procedures that do not involve informal influence and in-groups. Clear definitions of jobs and adequate resourcing of staff to undertake their work.

Children's Rights

Rights of children articulated and acted upon. Children and young people listened to and respected. User-friendly complaints procedures in place. Encouragement for children to discuss their hopes and feelings in a non-judgmental environment, where their concerns will be taken seriously and they will not be victimized for speaking out. Sex education and protective behaviors training provided; pornography banned. Permission for children to discuss sex as part of healthy development. Anti-oppressive environment: a non-sexist and non-racist culture that condemns abuse on grounds of difference.

BASIC PRINCIPLES OF GOOD SELECTION

More than a set of procedures, good staff selection practice is about a set of principles that embody particular attitudes to the task. If we achieved these basic principles, we would go a long way towards eliminating selection errors and the risk of abuse that follows such errors.

Focus on Quality, Not Abuse Prevention

> Aiming for the optimal is the most effective way of preventing systems abuse and so avoiding harm to children . . . it is not sufficient simply to avoid harm to children and to say what should not happen. It is also important to have a clear conception of positive end-point goals. (Cashmore, Dolby, & McGregor, 1994, p. 11)

Individuals with abusive tendencies are looking for opportunities where criteria for employment are not clearly identified and thus where they can simulate a vague image of a caring individual. Setting clear selection standards such as relevant training, experience, and job knowledge will rule out this opportunity for many of these individuals. The provision of information about agency standards and policies is also a part of this quality orientation. Large organizations need to find ways to ensure consistency of practice across the various program areas.

Practice Deterrence and Promotion of the Aware Culture

> Some of our smart paedophiles would sail through all the best-known selection procedures . . . (Platt, 1994)

Using good selection processes will deny entry to some abusive individuals. Others will need to be deterred. Remember that a preferential abuser is looking for a clear opportunity to enter an unaware environment. Making it clear from the beginning of the recruitment phase that your organization is not one of these will aid the deterrence process. Details of how to do this appear throughout this handbook.

Allow Time

> Spend time and lots of it. (Peters, 1988, p. 379)

You cannot improve your selection practice if you do not have reasonable time to devote to it. Persuade the organization of the value of putting in time here by looking at examples where avoidable mistakes have been made, and what it has cost in time, money, and human misery.

Train Managers in Staff Selection

There is a lot to learn in this field that cannot be written in to one small handbook. This is not a job for amateurs. Line managers who routinely select staff need to attend a short course that teaches the skills of staff selection. These are readily available through tertiary institutions and private training providers.

Draw on Personnel Knowledge

> There seems to be no other area of managerial practice where a large academic research literature has been as systematically ignored as it has been in the area of employee selection. (Dreher & Maurer, 1989, p. 249)

There is plenty of well-founded research to guide better practice. We need to use it if we are to select the best staff and minimize the risk of child abuse in human services programs. The ideas in this handbook are all based on solid personnel research.

Distrust Conventional Wisdom

The two most commonly used methods of staff selection–the selection interview and the reference check–are also among the least reliable. So is the old myth that it is all a matter of "gut feeling." We need more than gut feelings if we are to reduce the selection errors of the past. Intuition is important, but needs to be harnessed and justified by good practice.

Use Multiple Indicators of Suitability

Because we are using such unreliable selection tools, we need more than one way of assessing applicants' skills. The interview alone is definitely not enough. This handbook suggests some other options to add to the process.

Don't Confuse Screening Devices with Selection Devices

The reference check and the criminal records check are the usual problems here. Reference checks used to confirm interview impressions give us little independent information about the applicant. A criminal records check *must* be done on every prospective new staff member to ensure that he or she is not a convicted offender. However, it will not tell us anything about the suitability of an applicant for a job or even whether they are criminally inclined. Most abuse and offending goes undetected by the law. Screening devices are applied on a pass/fail basis only. They include criminal records, identity, qualifications, and suitable work history. They do not qualify a person for a job.

Selection methods should be applied to more than one applicant and treated independently of each other. More information can be gained by using the reference check as a selection tool than as a pass/fail screen. For example, references should be conducted on all applicants who seem to meet selection criteria in the interview. While this takes a little longer, it will improve selection decisions.

Use Similar Standards for Volunteer Selection

Volunteerism presents opportunities for abusers, because agencies often set vague, implicit standards about what sort of a person they are seeking to recruit, which tend to amount to "a nice person." Standards need to be set in similar ways to those for staff by writing volunteer job descriptions and key performance indicators, by careful selection, and follow up with induction, supervision, and support. Agencies need to be able to provide regular supervision, support and training for volunteers, or such programs may become key opportunities for abuse. Volunteer Centers in each state may be able to assist with guidelines for working with volunteers.

Utilize Equal Employment Opportunity (EEO) Principles

The application of EEO guidelines actually assists in making an accurate selection decision by excluding factors that are not job-relevant. All relevant material can be asked for in the application form or interview, providing it is phrased so as to make its job relevance clear (See Appendix A). The difficulty arises when assumptions are made as to what personal circumstances may affect job performance. For example, in the past we had the concern that women would take more time off to care for sick children than men. In fact, statistics have shown women to be more reliable in work attendance than men.

There are some work situations where it may be genuinely job-relevant to appoint a worker of a particular gender or culture. EEO exemptions are available for some such situations.

Use Induction and Socialization to Follow Up Selection

> The induction process is of critical importance to the new worker and deserves considerable attention by the organization. The impressions generated upon entry into the agency are lasting ones, and it is to the agency's advantage that orientation programs be positive experiences. (Pecora & Austin, 1987, p. 117)

This is an important further opportunity for deterring the potential abuser by reinforcing aware culture. Staff are at their most receptive in the early days and weeks on the job. Attention paid to teaching the job and reinforcing good practice and an aware culture is time well spent. The staff member who elects to leave suddenly at an early stage should not necessarily be discouraged; they may have identified their mismatch to the job better than we have. Agencies thus minimize their investment in the induction/socialization period at their own cost.

Train, Support and Supervise Staff

Maintaining a good staff who will provide quality service and not abuse children is not just a matter of selecting the right people and avoiding selecting an abuser. Situational abuse occurs when staff are not adequately supported, supervised and trained. It is critical to maintain good management and support once staff are on board.

Maintain an Open Culture

> Incidents or situations of harm to a child in care need to be viewed, and responded to, not as an abusive action by an individual but as a

> breach or dereliction of duty at individual, program and agency levels. (Forward, 1995, p. 22-23)

> One of the main dangers of institutions such as residential care establishments is their tendency to become closed and resistant to scrutiny by the general community. (Cashmore, Dolby, & McGregor, 1994, p. 63)

Investigations of abuse in institutions have repeatedly shown that the abuse was known to more than one person long before it was finally stopped (Beedell & Clough, 1992). Maintaining an open culture is a matter of leadership and policy and of the involvement of outsiders in management and the program.

RECRUITMENT

We would like to think that our selection processes could be so good as to reliably identify and eliminate the application of a child abuser. No such luck. However, we may not always see the key opportunity available before the selection stage to deter the abuser from even applying. Successfully done, we may never be aware that the deterrence took place. Below are some of the ways the recruitment phase can be used to promote quality and deter the abuser (see Figure 1).

Job Descriptions

Research indicates that the selection problems begin when organizations are not clear about the job itself and what is necessary to perform it. This is a significant opportunity for the preferential abuser to bluff his way. There are a variety of models for a job description. One such appears in Appendix C. Keep the job description clear, specific, brief, and up to date.

Key Performance Indicators

You need to be quite clear before you advertize as to what are your essential and what are your desirable criteria. After the interviews is late to debate whether a degree or diploma is necessary, how much experience and of what sort the person needs or whether he or she needs to be available for out-of-hours work. Key performance indicators need to be

FIGURE 1. A Model of Recruitment, Selection and Support

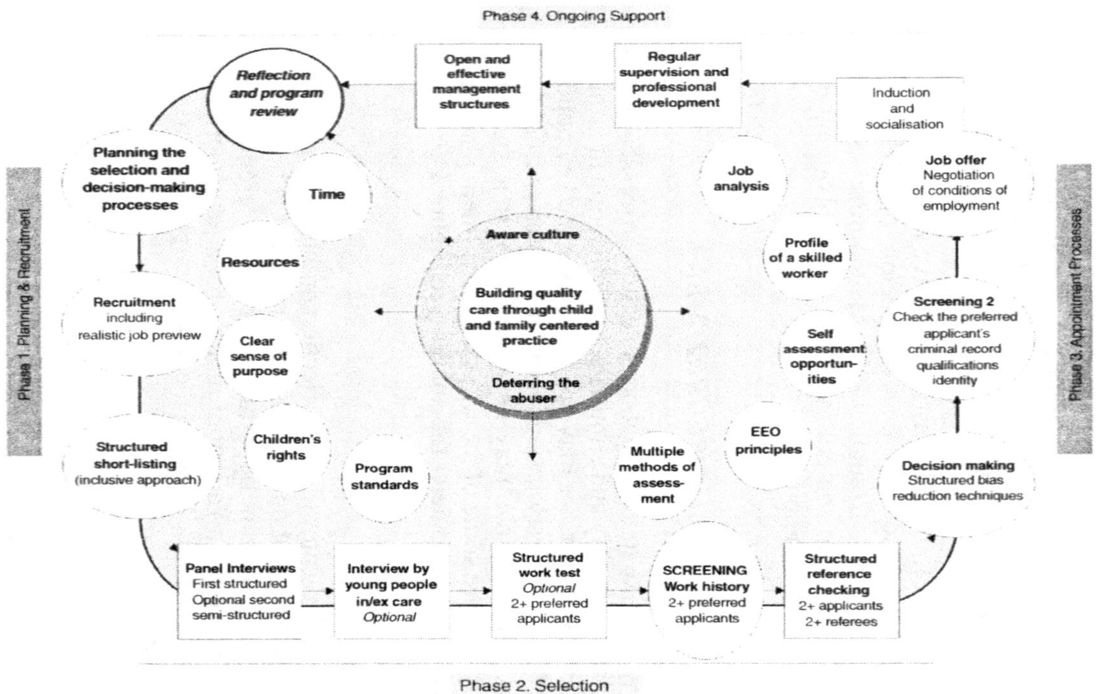

detailed on the bottom of the job description so that applicants can self-assess and screen themselves for you. Clear key performance indicators will eliminate some potential abusers who cannot meet them. An example appears in Appendix C.

Self-Assessment and Deterring the Abuser at the Outset

We do know that there are a number of dimensions on which people can assess themselves better than others can assess them. Among these is their ability and job performance (Fletcher, 1985). We also know that people's willingness to accurately self-assess is highly dependant upon the situation. In a job interview, it is probably at its lowest: applicants are there to sell themselves, not to be fully honest about their profile of strengths and weaknesses! At home, when first toying with a job application, motivation to self-assess may be much higher. We want to harness this motivation to assist us with the task of selection. Linked to this, we want to assist the abuser to assess for himself that he would be poorly matched to our work environment. This can be done by the sort of information we put in front of potential applicants.

Realistic Job Previews (RJPs)

A Realistic Job Preview (RJP) that stresses both the positive and negative aspects of the job has been found to set job expectations at realistic levels, to improve job satisfaction, and reduce staff turnover (Wanous, 1982). It will not reduce the flow of highly capable applicants. We also know that a RJP used early in the recruitment process is likely to be of more value than one used later. When an individual has set their mind on a course of action, they tend to seek only information that confirms their choice (Gardner, Foo, & Hesketh, 1995). At the inquiry stage is then the best time for giving realistic information. The RJP can then assist applicants to self-assess suitability for a job and give another opportunity to deter the would-be abuser.

Below are some ways of providing realistic job previews.

Information Packages

An inclusive information package might include the job description and key performance indicators, a program description, and the organization's relevant brochure(s) and key policies. There may be an information booklet for new staff. This may be an area in which there is some work to be done. In a child-focused service, key policies might be child discipline, children's rights, and complaints procedures. Brochures and policy statements between them should detail the agency mission and expectations of practice. They should also make it clear that the agency has an aware culture and promotes human rights, in particular, children's rights. A clear, consistent message in these documents sets a standard and style of practice expected and makes it clear that this is an environment in which a child abuser will have difficulty achieving his ends.

> *Time spent on preparing a detailed package of program materials that promote the agency's interest in quality care, alertness to the possibility of child abuse, and measures that are in place to counteract abuse, may be the single most effective step you can take to minimize the risk of abuse within your program.*

Information Sessions

Many agencies invite prospective staff to an information session. This is an opportunity for both a Realistic Job Preview and further work on promoting agency culture and deterring the potential abuser. Where a number of staff are being recruited at once this is strongly recommended. Applicants should be asked to hold their application until they have attended such a session. An information session could include discussion with staff already on the job, watching a video on the program, or a program visit.

Application Forms

A standard application form has a series of advantages. It ensures that applicants provide a detailed work history, which is important for identifying if there have been performance problems in the past. It also allows for negotiating appropriate references with the applicant (see below). The application form gives an opportunity to ask about any criminal record and for permission to undertake a criminal records check. Applicants can be encouraged to detail job-relevant training and experience–formal and informal. It should include a signed declaration that all the information is true and correct. This makes for clear process in dealing with any problems of honesty that are identified later.

While some applicants will give all this information in a letter or curriculum vitae, others will forget, not be aware of what is required, "fudge," or lie. Where the job is not a professional one, an application form also assists the less literate but able worker to present their case for employment.

The application form becomes the basis for short-listing.

Short-Listing

With identified key performance criteria and a standard application form, as well as possibly a curriculum vitae and covering letter, short-listing becomes a straightforward, objective process. A grid needs to be developed outlining essential and desirable qualifications and experience. A category should be included for unusual but relevant experience. A sample grid is included in Appendix C.

Inclusiveness in Recruitment

If we are to appoint the best possible applicant and avoid recruiting an abuser, we need to choose from the widest possible field. Unless the numbers of applicants meeting all essential criteria are overwhelming, all of these should be listed for interview. The interview will quickly reduce numbers. We tend to overlook the possibility of missing a suitable applicant (Type 2 error) because we are so focused on not appointing the wrong person (Type 1 error) (Anderson & Shackleton, 1993, p. 61). This will be a problem if no suitable applicant emerges from the interview process.

THE EMPLOYMENT INTERVIEW

The interview is the commonest and almost universally used selection device. Sometimes it is used on its own, sometimes in conjunction with a reference check, and more rarely with other selection devices. "It is disturbing, then, to find that there is a vast research literature that points to its unreliability. Reviews of the selection interviewing research . . . have found that its popularity is not matched by its validity" (Wright, Lichtenfels, & Pursell, 1989, p. 191).

Fortunately, however, there has also been considerable research finding ways to improve the interview. The single most important method is by systematically structuring the interview–although not to the point of rigidity. A standard list of questions needs to be developed that relate closely to the job description and key selection criteria. Follow-up probing questions should be used to clarify responses, encourage the less articulate interviewee to elaborate on their skills, and to pick up on the specific experience of individuals. Probing questions should not be used to introduce red herrings or questions that violate Equal Employment Opportunity. (So asking about the book on their bedside table or who will pick up the children from school is out.) See below, Equal Employment Opportunity in the Interview.

Short courses are available in selection interviewing. Anyone whose job it is to interview for staff should have undergone such training.

Questioning Style

Open and Closed Questions

Closed questions invite a yes/no answer. They are useful for gaining factual information, but most of this should have been obtained via the application form and curriculum vitae.

> How many years did you work for the insurance company?

Open questions invite the applicant to tell you about their relevant experience and skills. They are more useful for the purpose of job interviewing.

> Can you please tell us about the skills and experience you have that you feel may have prepared you for this job?

> Can you tell us about your work on the village education project?

Leading Questions

Most of us think we wouldn't be so silly as to ask leading questions or questions that reveal the desired answer. Most of us still do. Who would say no to any of these questions?

> Would you describe yourself as a patient person?

> Do you see yourself as well-organized?

> Can you handle stress?

We need some more volunteers. Are you good at recruitment?

Interview Approaches

Two specific developments in interviewing techniques are useful approaches to improving selection interviews.

Situational Interviewing

This is the most familiar approach. It involves the development of scenario-type questions that are based upon examples of tasks that are part of the job. In developing situational questions, it is important to take some time and check that questions are neither obvious, nor tricky, or worded in such a way that the right answer is fed to the interviewer. Good situational questions are challenging to write. Sometimes clients of the service can give good ideas about useful mini-scenarios.

Behavioral Interviewing

The advocates of Behavioral Interviewing (or Patterned Behavioral Description Interviewing) maintain that situational questions tend to be easy to fake. What people say they would do and what they would really do are said to be two different things. These people claim that "the best prophet of the future is the past" (Janz, 1989). They suggest that it is much harder to fake an answer when asked to describe real life experiences from the past.

Examples of a behavioral questioning approach are:

> Could you tell me about a time when you were working with a child whom you took a dislike to? How did you handle the situation so that you could still do your job?

> Could you tell me about a time when you disagreed with a colleague about how to do something important? How did you resolve the issue?

Interviewees often find these questions difficult and may resort to giving situational answers. They might say:

> Oh, I don't usually get into conflict. I usually just discuss problems openly and we work it out.

Answers like this need to be gently probed for a real life experience. Interviewees need to be told these questions are quite difficult and that the panel can wait while they think of a suitable example. This is a challenging interviewing technique.

Examples of behavioral questions appear in Appendix A.

Other Areas for Interview Exploration

Job Knowledge Questions

The key selection criteria will have identified what professional or specialist knowledge must be brought to the job as opposed to what can be learned quickly at the outset. A few questions should then probe whether the applicant can give evidence of an appropriate level of mastery of key areas.

Attitudinal Questions

Suitable open questions that do not lead the answer need to be developed to test for attitudes.

> What are your thoughts about the most important aspects of running a development program?
>
> What do you see as the most important parts of being a team leader?
>
> If you could leave behind a couple of areas of good practice in this program, what would they be?
>
> What is the best way to work with underperforming staff?
>
> How important is textbook knowledge in a job like this?
>
> How would you create a work environment that would minimize the opportunity for child abuse?

Reinforcing Policy

Relevant policies could be sent out to applicants short-listed for interview. The interview then becomes a chance to test how thoroughly the applicant read them, and to invite their comments on them. In doing so, the agency reminds the applicant that they are serious about their policies and expect new staff to work within them. This is an important part of abuse prevention. Where "aware culture" policies are clearly articulated, a preferential abuser may decide that this program will present too many chances to get caught and go elsewhere.

Asking the Difficult Questions

If we cannot be confident about identifying an abuser in a job interview, then we need to focus as much on deterring an abuser (or encouraging them to self-select out) as on looking for indicators of abusive attitudes. Asking direct, challenging questions is designed for this end rather than with the expectation that abusive individuals will reveal themselves as such.

The model of questioning that focuses on deterrence includes such questions as:

> Have you ever worked anywhere where a colleague abused a child? What happened and how was it handled? What did you think of the way it was handled? Would you have handled it differently yourself?
>
> Are you aware of our policy about children's rights? What do you think of it? Can you see any problems with it?
>
> Have you thought about how you might feel if a child or young person lodged a complaint of abuse against you? How would you want such a complaint to be handled?
>
> What steps do you take to ensure that this is unlikely to happen to you?
>
> What are your views about touching children and young people? When might it be appropriate to comfort a child by putting an arm round them?
>
> When do you think this might be appropriate and when not appropriate to be alone with a child?
>
> Have you ever had a child or teenager make a sexual advance towards you? Why might this happen? What did you do, or what might you do?

> Do you think that children and young people need special friends and mentors at times? How might you be a mentor for a young person without getting too close?
>
> Have you ever abused a child? (Wait for a response.) What happened? What would you do if this situation arose again? We ask this question of all applicants, because we want them to be aware of the culture within which they will work. Vulnerable children such as those in our programs attract abusive people, and they find it difficult to tell people if they have been abused. That is why we have training sessions for both children and staff on abuse prevention, and complaints procedures that are designed to make it possible for children to speak out about abuse. When an allegation is made, we attempt to support staff, but we also listen carefully to the child. We would want to think about whether you would be comfortable working in an environment like this.

This is a challenging arena of interviewing. However, it may be the best chance to deter a preferential abuser–and begin to set parameters for a situational abuser–that we have at the present time (Waldron, personal communication, 1994).

Red Flags

The real risk here is the assumption that "you can pick them." Warning signs *can* be as obvious as the man who talks of being the friend to all the local kids, the one who takes them out and has an exceptional rapport with them. They can also be less clear. It might be overly smooth presentation or keenness to please. It might be poor communication skills, poor listening, or rapport. It might be none of these. It is our belief that the signs may not be clear and that a skilled pedophile may not be detected by "gut feel" or obvious warning signs. He may, in fact, simulate the profile of the sort of "sensitive new age guy" you had in mind for the job. He may, however, be ruled out as underqualified or because of soft signs of dishonesty or inappropriateness in other areas. It is likely that you will never know whether some of those you screen out carefully on clear job-related grounds were actually preferential abusers seeking entry into a program with unclear requirements of its staff.

Equal Employment Opportunity in the Interview

There is an acceptable way to ask for almost every item of job-relevant information. However, there is no guarantee that applicants will be honest, regardless of how the questions are asked. There is no need to know someone's age, marital status or sexual preference to determine if they can perform the job well. Examples of acceptable and unacceptable questions appear in Appendix B.

The Selection Panel

A selection panel offers support to the line manager in making a complex decision and offers the benefit of a range of perspectives. The blind spot of one panel member (which might even be a very experienced interviewer) may be counteracted by the insight of another. A slick presentation may impress one panel member and arouse warning signs in another. Remember the value of a selection panel lies in the *differences* of perceptions as well as the similarities.

- A good size selection panel is two or three people. Large panels can be intimidating. If political considerations dictate a bigger panel, five should definitely be a maximum.
- The ideal panel is balanced for gender, for example, a male and a female and, where possible, ethnic origin to minimize bias.
- The line manager should be on the panel. A front-line worker in a similar position can be an advantage because of their inside knowledge of the job. A third party might be someone outside of the employing organization who knows the field. This encourages openness in the assessment process.
- At least one person on the panel should have been trained in selection interviewing.
- Service clients have a valuable place in assisting with selection of staff. One may be on the selection panel or, better still, a small group could do their own interview. This is described below.

Involving the Clients in Staff Selection

Service users have been involved in staff selection in many organizations with programs for disabled people. This practice has been slower to filter into child welfare and other areas of human services.

Why Do It?

Client participation in program development and management is increasingly seen as both good practice and an issue of rights. There is also the potential to obtain a unique perspective on how applicants actually relate to clients that may be difficult for management to achieve. Further, there may be a deterrent message in an approach like this that signals the empowering of children and young people within programs set up for them.

> The young people contributed something valuable . . . they brought experience and insights which could not have been matched within any conventional interviewing panel. They provided the employing agency with a critical opportunity to observe how well the candidates actually interacted and communicated with young people . . . An additional advantage in involving young people in this way is the message it gives to candidates about the employing agency. Hopefully, it will introduce an element of self-selection for those who are not prepared to work in partnership with young people, or, worse, those who have ulterior motives in seeking this kind of work. (Lindsay & Rayner, 1993, p. 25)

Implementation

The most effective and empowering way to do this is to arrange, with training and support, for young people (or other clients) to form a small selection panel of their own. The group members give each other confidence and staff/client power differentials are minimized. It has been the experience of staff who have assisted young people in this process that even the most challenging young people have taken these unusual responsibilities seriously and conducted their interviews with care and respect for applicants and the agency. The final selection decision remains, of course, with the employing agency.

Involving young people–or service users of any age and situation–in staff selection can bring unexpected benefits in a number of ways. However, in order to work well it needs to be introduced into a program that already has children's rights recognized and implemented in a variety of other ways. An additional investment of time and energy is required if this process is to work well.

Making Decisions

We know that interviewers are very poor at processing information from the interview and making accurate decisions. "Interviewers are the major source of error, being prone to a variety of disfunctions in their information-processing strategies" (Anderson & Shackleton, 1993, p. 68). They also have the capacity to bias each other and thus minimize the value of having a panel of people who can contribute their different perspectives. It is easy to pick the outstanding applicant; the challenge lies in making a good decision when there is no outstanding applicant.

Common Interviewer Biases

Anderson and Shackleton (1993) list the twelve major dysfunctions in interviewer decision-making. These are:

1. Expectancy effect–Interviewers form an expectancy of the candidate based on documented biographical information that strongly affects their final decision.
2. Confirmatory information-seeking bias–Interviewers actively seek information to confirm their initial impressions.
3. Primacy effect–Interviewers form impressions of applicants very early on in the interview.
4. Stereotyping and prototyping–Interviewers possess notions of stereotypical and prototypical ideal job holders and screen applicants against these notions.
5. Halo/horns effect–Interviewers interpret information and rate applicants in either a generally positive or generally negative manner.
6. Contrast and quota effect–Interviewers' decisions are affected by decisions on earlier applicants and pre-set employment quotas.
7. Negative information bias–Interviewers' decisions are influenced significantly more by negative information than by positive information.
8. Similar-to-me effect–Interviewers select applicants similar to themselves in biographical background, personality and attitudes.
9. Personal liking bias–Interviewers favor applicants whom they like personally.

10. Information overload and selective attention–Interviewers have too much information to cope with and so attend to only a fraction of the available data.
11. Fundamental attrition error–Interviewers incorrectly attribute the cause of applicant behavior at interview to their personality rather than to situational constraints and demands.
12. Temporal extension–Interviewers "temporarily extend" applicant behavior at interview to infer longer term emotional states and personality traits. (pp. 56-63)

These biases should be discussed with the panel in the initial briefing and strategies devised to counter them. For example, the decision-making process at the end might include some discussion of when panel members were aware of their own or each other's biases.

Other ways of counteracting bias are:

- Interviewing for a maximum of one-half day (reducing information overload and selective attention).
- Once the short list is made, paying little attention to the written application or preconceived ideas about the applicant (counteracting expectancy effect, confirmatory information-seeking bias).
- Make the interviews of reasonable length. There is some evidence to suggest that this may mitigate against premature decision-making or primacy effect.
- Consciously question myths and stereotypes in yourself and each other (counteracting stereotyping and prototyping, personal liking).

Use of Rating Scales

A powerful form of group bias sets in as the interviewee closes the door behind them. Panel members look at each other and convey, verbally and non-verbally, their impressions, particularly if strongly positive or negative. In that moment, a more influential panel member may have influenced others so that differing impressions may be suppressed or revised. *(What was I thinking? Of course he is OK/unsuitable. She should know, she's done this for a long time.)*

It is the view of experts on this subject that group consensus should definitely not be used to make the selection decision (Anderson, 1994; Fletcher, 1994). Rating scales should be filled in before the panel exchange views, grimaces, grins, etc. Discussion should then focus on explaining the reasons for the ratings given and hearing each other's perspectives before there is any attempt to reach a joint decision. An example of a rating scale for selection interviewing appears in Appendix C.

Still Not Sure?

Every employment decision is an important one. That feeling of uncertainty may be your only clue that the person in front of you is not the one for the job–or is a potential abuser. Use your gut feeling to good, systematic ends and bring them back for a second interview or negotiate for another referee or a work test (see next section). The reason for your uncertainty may come clear one way or another with more information.

REFERENCE CHECKS

Reference checks have a few things in common with selection interviews:

- almost everyone uses them,
- research has shown them to be extremely unreliable (Muchinsky, 1979; Dobson, 1989), and
- nobody believes this.

Fortunately, authorities on the reference check have also given us some clues as to what to do to improve them.

Why are they so unreliable? Because the applicant selects them for their capacity to sell the strengths of the applicant. Thus, the referees given may not always be those who know the applicant's work the best, or those who are able to be objective in their views. Referees are sometimes personal friends made in the workplace. Conversely, a referee may be a current supervisor who sees the person as a poor performer and/or dislikes the person, and wants to "sell" them to someone else!

Sometimes an applicant struggles to find an appropriate referee through no fault of their own. Accepting a poor or naive choice of referees may not give us the information we need. We need to continue to do reference checks–because it is seen as good practice, and we open ourselves to litigation if we don't. But we must improve practice if they are to tell us anything useful.

Again, take time. You cannot afford to make a mistake. Don't rush through the references to confirm your interview decision. Time spent here is time well spent, even if it means not having a staff member for another week.

What can we do differently? The first and most important improvement is the same as for the selection interview. Structure your approach carefully and eliminate the *ad hoc* nature of reference checking of the past.

Structuring the Reference Check

- One person (usually the line manager) should do all the reference checks. This improves consistency and confidentiality.
- Use a standard list of questions that is asked of every referee. Use customized follow-up questions as appropriate to the applicant and the situation.
- Document the reference check as it is being taken, on a form that lists each question and has room for the answer underneath (this is hard work). A proforma appears in Appendix C.
- Always ask first how long the referee has known the person and in what capacity–including whether they are personal friends.
- Ask specifically about both skills, and areas that need development, in separate questions.
- Ask other questions that are related specifically to the key performance indicators.
- Ask about the person's receptivity to supervision and direction.
- Always ask specifically whether the referee is aware that the person has ever abused a child or behaved in an unprofessional way. (This question may surprise the referee, but will rarely be viewed as inappropriate.)
- Ask the referee how strongly they would recommend the applicant, e.g., not at all, with reservations, recommend, strongly recommend, don't know, not willing to say.
- Follow up on pauses and hesitations. If necessary, remind the referee of your Duty of Care to make suitable appointments.

How Many References?

- Try to do references for more than one preferred applicant. You are aiming to make a selection, not confirm your preconceived ideas from the interview. Use the reference check as an independent selection tool, not a screening device.

- Do at least two references for each applicant. If there are any areas of concern and you are still considering appointing the person, ask for more referees to check these out specifically. If you know someone who may be able to give a relevant perspective, ask the applicant for permission to ring them.
- If you are not satisfied that appropriate referees can recommend the applicant or know his/her work well enough, negotiate with the applicant for other referees, or do not appoint him/her.

Other Considerations

- Use the application form to collect a detailed work history, then check referees given against the work history. If the referees are not their most recent supervisors, ask why. Hear both sides of the story if there has been a clash, and if necessary ask to speak to someone else who could comment impartially if the story is difficult to resolve. Insist on speaking to the appropriate referees regardless of the applicant's story, and make your own judgement.
- Try to avoid using informal networks. As well as being unethical, they may give you biased personal perspectives. Negotiate with your applicant for appropriate referees. If you want to speak to another person about him/her, tell the applicant first.
- Always ask the referee if they are in private when you call and can spare 10-15 minutes right then. Many will ring you back if given the chance, and then you have their full attention. Make sure you are also in private when you speak to them.
- Always ring the most appropriate work-based referees, wherever they are. Do not accept personal referees unless there is a genuine reason why two work-based referees cannot be given (e.g., a new graduate). Don't use the most convenient ones. Be willing to make national and international calls.
- Attempt some evaluation of the referee where possible. How well do they know the applicant's work? Do they seem overly positive or negative? How experienced are they in the field?

Confidentiality and Storage

Remember that most references are given in confidence. If personnel files are open to staff perusal on request, a separate file should be created for references. This file should be kept it in a locked filing cabinet to which staff do not have access.

ALTERNATIVE METHODS OF SELECTION

There is now an overwhelming body of opinion among those who work in human services fields that the most effective way to assess a person's competence is through some form of work test or job tryout (Cohen & Gump, 1984; Denholm, 1988). The following quotations came from a review of recruitment and selection processes in the United Kingdom. (This review was prompted by a particularly appalling series of abuses of children in care by Frank Beck, a man who succeeded in gaining more than one position in residential care even after abuses were disclosed in the first position.)

> We consider that selection processes which most closely simulate the actual experience of working in a post are the most effective. We recognize that effective simulation of work in a children's home will be extremely difficult to achieve. However, it should be possible to simulate the *environment* in the home, and to consider how applicants respond to it. (United Kingdom Department of Health, 1992, p. 49)

> The view that the most reliable method of selection was work simulations came from every angle. (Davis, personal communication, 1994)

Work tests or tryouts are not always easy to set up. Depending on the nature of the program, possibilities could include:

- Employment in a casual capacity for a limited number of days or shifts on a mutual assessment basis;
- Recruitment from a pool of casual or part-time staff;
- An extended visit to the program involving meeting other staff and program clients, possibly followed by an interview and/or a written response to a series of related questions. Depending on the program, the applicant might be able to undertake a nominated task during the visit, perhaps working with a client or staff member;
- Viewing of audiotaped behavioral vignettes from work on the program and responding to these either verbally or in writing;

- Oral and/or written response to vignettes presented on paper.

Work tests and exercises need careful and fair assessment like any other selection method. They should be standardized as much as possible. A rating scale like the one used for the selection interview would be desirable. The same staff, preferably the line manager, should conduct all the work tests for the different applicants.

Program clients may have valuable feedback on the suitability of the applicant. They may be able to detect nuances of behavior that escape staff. Their involvement in a program visit may be a useful way to collect this additional perspective.

It may be practical to offer a work test only to a small group of applicants who have already been interviewed.

PSYCHOLOGICAL TESTING

For many years practitioners and researchers have sought to find a more objective and "scientific" way to test for child abuse potential. The idea of such a screening device is an attractive one. At the present time, we are bound for disappointment here. A recent comprehensive review of psychological tests used in human services staff selection revealed that there is no test in existence that has yet been successfully validated as being able to identify abusive staff (Kiraly, 1988).

Psychological testing in personnel selection is also big business. Several companies in Australia and overseas have indicated their interest in selling their products to human services agencies with confident undertakings about their value in detecting potential abusers.

There is also a risk that psychological tests may be used as a "magic solution" to the question of pedophile screening, leading to a false sense of security, and blinding agencies to the ever-present risk that a pedophile may have entered their employ. The use of tests may also divert agencies from improving their overall staff selection practices.

Should your agency decide to go down this path, remember:

- Some of the tests that are in use in the personnel selection industry are more reputable than others. All must be administered by a qualified psychologist.
- Psychological testing should always be an additional process rather than a substitute for other good practice.

- In using psychological tests, Equal Employment Opportunity issues need to be kept in mind. The test should in some way be validated for the purpose to which it is to be put.

PRE-EMPLOYMENT CHECKS

Based upon the bitter experience of agencies in the past, we now know that a series of pre-employment checks are a necessary part of good selection practice. Most of them have been mandatory in local child welfare services for some years.

Pre-employment checks are screening devices, not selection tests. None of them qualify a person for a job, but failure on any one should normally rule out the appointment on honesty grounds if no other.

Identity

The rare but spectacularly awful incidents of child abuse in employment are often associated with false identity. You cannot afford to take the risk. Check two forms of identity, one with a photo. A passport or drivers license and an original birth certificate are a good combination. If you are in any doubt, don't dismiss your concerns. Take the identification to your line manager. Someone who is going to deceive in this way may be a smooth and convincing operator who can apparently easily dismiss some difference in the photo from present-day appearance.

Qualifications

Again, the person who claims to have a degree but does not is a rare one, but it has happened. More frequently, a curriculum vitae is written in such a way to disguise the fact that a course of study is incomplete. This may not matter, but you need to know both what studies the applicant has done, and whether they are honest about their credentials and other things.

You need to see the original copy of their results, or their degree or diploma certificate. If they need to bring in the whole frame, so be it!

Driver's License

If staff are to drive as part of their duties, you must see this. Check for any endorsements or whether the license is probationary. These may not matter, but you need to know.

Work History

This is critical: it is the area in which people are most likely to "fudge" their background. Check the application form and/or curriculum vitae to see if months as well as years in previous employment are listed. 1992-1993 can mean a summer job of six weeks.

The use of an application form that asks for a detailed work history (dates, employing organization and nature of work) is useful here (See Appendix C). Probe for details if you are not clear. Check with referees to verify.

Criminal Records Check

A criminal records check must be done for every applicant for work in human services or humanitarian aid, whether paid or voluntary. However, this is not quite as straightforward as it looks.

> An estimated 4% of all offences committed result in a criminal conviction. (United Kingdom Department of Health, 1992, p. 72)

> Less than 1% of people who engage in acts of child molestation have a criminal records history. (Moriarty, 1990, p. 60)

Clearly, a negative criminal record tells us nothing about whether the person is an offender against children or the community.

Why Do It Then?

In the past, people have been appointed to positions with criminal records that were unknown to the employer. We cannot take that chance. Further, the systematic use of criminal records checks may be acting as a deterrent to a small group of convicted offenders to whom this field will no longer be open. We are simply expected to do this check and render ourselves liable if we do not.

While it will be rare to pick up a record of conviction against children now that criminal records checks are so widespread, from time to time a record of other offences will be identified. These will require judgement as to whether they constitute a reason not to employ. See below.

The real danger of using criminal records checks lies in the assumption that a negative criminal record means that the person is fit for employment in human services. In an emergency, some agencies in the past have done a telephone police check and then employed someone with minimal selection procedures. This is dangerous practice.

> I believe that criminal history check requirements contribute to a lowering, rather than raising, of our standards for entry into the field of child care. If you don't have a criminal record, then you meet the minimum qualifications to work with children. (Carter, 1986, p. 31)

Guidelines for Implementation

- Always do a criminal records check, and never count on it to tell you anything about the applicant's suitability for the job. It is a screen, not a selection device.
- The best place to start this process is by using an application form that asks applicants to declare any criminal history and give signed consent for a criminal records check to be undertaken. If the check then reveals anything that has not been declared, you may have a dishonesty problem on your hands.
- A judgement needs to be made as to what offences render a person unsuitable for employment. The prime area of concern is, of course, child abuse. An undeclared criminal record of any sort should be grounds for rejection. So should an extended criminal history of any kind, even if minor. Other areas that may be of concern are:

  Assault;

  Driving offences, such as drunk or dangerous driving, particularly if driving is part of the job;

  Dishonesty offences;

  Substance abuse offences.

It is possible that any of these may be single events, minor, and/or from long ago, and include mitigating circumstances. However, offences in one area may be the only clue to problems in another, e.g., poor self-control, dishonesty, etc. When in doubt, don't employ.

- A positive criminal record should be discussed with the applicant, together with the decision the employer has taken regarding it, and reasons. The reasons should be documented for future reference.
- Overseas applicants present some challenges. There have been rare but serious incidents of pedophiles arriving from overseas and gaining access to employment because their criminal record was unknown. It is important to find some way to check overseas records. This could be via the reference of a previous employer, followed up in writing. This should be done by direct communication with the referee, not by a written reference supplied by the applicant.

Privacy and Confidentiality

- Check on the person you wish to employ, after all selection processes, including the reference checks, are complete.
- The only person in an organization to handle criminal records checks should be the human resources manager or the line manager. Forms should be returned from the police unopened and filed in a separate file in a secure place. They should not be stored on personnel files.

DOCUMENTATION

Documentation is important to demonstrate that the selection decision was fair and reasonable and in case of a challenge to the decision. We don't have time for onerous recording, and it does not need to be. The documentation should involve a brief report in three sections:

- One briefly describing the process used;
- A second consisting of proformas used in the process (not completed);
- A third is a confidential section to be destroyed after a year, including the applications and ratings of each short-listed applicant.

A simple report format appears in Appendix D.

Storage of Information

The application and curriculum vitae should be kept on the person's personnel file. The reference check records and criminal records check should be kept in two separate files dedicated to these purposes. All this information should be kept in secure files.

Destruction of Confidential Material

The line manager or human resources manager should take responsibility for destroying all copies of job applications and other confidential material that is no longer needed.

STAFF SUPPORT AND MANAGEMENT

Induction and Socialization

As important to good staffing as a good selection process is the induction/socialization process that should commence straight after appointment (Anderson, 1994). This is *the* key opportunity to minimize the risk of abusive behavior by teaching the concept of the aware culture in all its aspects and modelling it to newcomers.

> Information about the unit's role and scope provides the worker with a better perspective of the organization's mission . . . There will probably be few other opportunities for a supervisor to capture the worker's openness and receptivity to acquiring a positive attitude toward his or her job. (Pecora & Austin, 1987, p. 119)

> The initial recruitment process is only the start. If a programme of induction is to be of benefit it . . . should seek to share the ethos of the organization and to assist in the future development of both the individual and the organization. (National Children's Bureau, 1994, p. 2)

Socialization is much more than showing a new worker the ropes and giving practical information about the new work-place. It includes these aspects, but goes beyond them to use the opportunity to imbue in the new employee the values, attitudes, and expectations of the agency in relation to its work with children, young people and their families. This is the opportunity to provide support and guidance to the new worker, to make them feel comfortable, to provide whatever information and resources they need to learn the details of their new job, and to inculcate the professional standards and expectations of the agency with regard to the way the job is performed.

> [Socialization means] to learn the attitudes, standards, values and patterns of behavior that are expected by the organization and its management. [It] serves several purposes. It reduces the worker's anxiety by familiarizing him/her with what is expected in terms of attitudes, values and behaviors. It helps ensure consistent and predictable behavior by moulding the employee's attitudes and values to those of the employer. It reduces the need for policies, procedures and rules, to the extent that employees know how to act–and do so. And by making the new employee feel like "one of the family" it can increase the person's commitment to the organization, and thus may boost morale and lead to higher performance . . . (Dressler, 1988, p. 235)

Components of Induction

The Induction Kit

This should be available to the new staff member on the first day. It should include basic information such as staff lists, organizational chart, agency brochures and mission statement, the program description, key policy statements, and other administrative material as necessary.

Formal Induction Session

The agency should conduct a formal induction session every few months for staff who have come on board recently. Again, this provides an opportunity to reinforce agency ethos and the aware culture.

Site-Based Induction

The induction process needs to be intensive in the early phase and followed up over the ensuing weeks and months.

Link to Ongoing Supervision

Regular supervision should be established from the first week, initially on a weekly basis, with frequent informal, "responsive" supervision in between.

Supervision and Support

A lack of regular, formal supervision oriented towards quality practice has been a backdrop to much abusive practice. Management either did not know–or chose not to know–what was going on. Regular, formal supervision is a hallmark of good human services practice. It is the main vehicle of both support to staff and their accountability. It is an essential, time-consuming, and skilled process. Supervisors need to be trained in this complex skill.

Supervision sessions should be briefly minuted by the supervisor and a copy given to the staff member. This allows for issues to be followed up and decisions carried through to completion or resolution rather than forgotten or misconstrued by one party or the other.

Initial weekly supervision may gradually move to fortnightly or thrice-weekly as the staff member learns the job and becomes more independent. Supervision in human services should never drop below this frequency. Between formal sessions, staff need *ad hoc* responsive supervision. Access to responsive supervision in emergency or unusual circumstances should be available 24 hour per day in any program that has an after-hours component. The line supervisor should carry a pager for this purpose.

Supervision needs to address the administrative, learning, and support needs of the staff member. It is not enough to go through the motions for either staff member or line manager. The staff member needs the constant support of the supervisor, assistance to identify training needs and access them, and assistance to get to the bottom of any problems on the job or difficulties in performance. These should be addressed quickly–not left for a future performance appraisal.

Difficulties that develop in the supervisory relationship need to be tackled and not avoided by allowing supervision to become irregular or perfunctory. Occasionally this may necessitate the involvement of the supervisor's line manager or another third party.

Soft Signs of Abusive Practice

A predilection towards abuse may be picked up in supervision in one form or another. The staff member may give mixed message, or appear reluctant to be supervised or follow through on tasks. There may be soft signs of dishonesty in other areas such as money or time management. Vague, grey areas in relation to professional boundaries may be evident either from the person him/herself or by comments from other staff.

These should never be avoided through fear of making a false accusation. Rather, they should be raised as they have been reported and the issue of possible misperceptions acknowledged. Good practice standards, which reduce the likelihood of misperceptions, can then be reinforced. Issues like this should be carefully monitored, as they may be the only signs available to management that abuse is taking place, or is likely to. The staff member who is naive but innocent of abuse needs to be taught appropriate; the would-be abuser needs to be warned. When tackling issues in the "grey area," you may not be clear for some time which you are doing. This only makes it more important to be vigilant about your support, monitoring and limit-setting.

Training

> At worst it is irresponsible, and at best naive of agencies to believe that staffing residential programs with inexperienced, untrained and/or undertrained staff will somehow benefit clients. (Murphy, 1994, p. 32)

Residential child care is a field that has struggled for recognition of the skill level required to provide quality care and to avoid child abuse in its many forms. Other areas of human service practice suffer the same problems to varying degrees. In a field where resources are always limited, it is sometimes tempting to assume that a new staff member comes fully qualified and needs little in the way of further training.

In-service training is an investment for an agency. The creation of a learning environment in the work-place is a key component of delivering quality service and preventing child abuse. Training has the capacity to:

- set and maintain standards of work practice and teach how to maintain these standards;
- protect the safety and well-being of children and young people;
- reduce the incidents of abusive practice by preventing mistakes;
- bring new ideas and practice to staff;
- improve job performance and staff satisfaction and morale, leading to happier and more committed staff;
- make more effective use of limited resources;
- skill staff to take on new challenges. (United Kingdom Department of Health, 1992, VCOSS, 1993)

Training has the capacity to address some performance problems and potential abuse issues, particularly for the potential situational abuser. However, not all performance problems will be addressed by training. When identified as a means of improving problematic performance, and particularly when there is concern about potential abuse, the supervisor needs to pick up on the identified issues as well and follow them through.

References

A.B., & Y.Z. (pseud.) (1994, July 12). *Rights for young people.* Paper presented at the Residential Child Care: Into the Next Century. Day Conference run by the National Children's Bureau of the United Kingdom (NCB-UK), London, UK.

Australian Association of Young People in Care. (1994). Bill of rights. *Illusion Free Zone*, 8.

Ainsworth, F., & Small, R. W. (1994). Family centred group care practice: Concept and implementation. *Children Australia, 19*(4), 22-24.

American Psychological Association. (1977). Ethical standards of psychologists. Washington, DC: American Psychological Association.

American Psychological Association. (1980). Principles for the validation and use of personnel selection procedures: (2nd ed.). Washington, DC: American Psychological Association.

Anderson, M., & Shackleton, V. (1993). *Successful selection interviewing.* Oxford: Blackwell.

Anderson, N. R. (1992). Eight decades of employment interview research: A retrospective meta-review and prospective commentary. *European Work and Organizational Psychologist, 2*(1), 1-32.

Arvey, R. D. (1979). Unfair discrimination in the employment interview: Legal and psychological aspects. *Psychological Bulletin, 86*, 736-765.

Arvey, R. D. (1986). Commentary: General ability in employment–A discussion. *Journal of Vocational Behaviour, 29*, 415-420.

Arvey, R., & Campion, J. (1982). The employment interview: A summary and review of recent research. *Personnel Psychology, 35*, 291-322.

Association of Child Welfare Agencies. (1972, October). *Focus on children when families break down.* Paper presented at the Association of Child Welfare Agencies Conference, Consumer Session.

Australia. (1975). Racial discrimination act.

Australia. (1984). Sex discrimination act.

Australia. (1986). Human rights and equal opportunity commission act.

Australia. (1992). Disability discrimination act.

Australian Association of Young People in Care. (1994). *Illusion Free Zone, the Conference Edition.* Brisbane: New Color Process.

Barrett, G. V., & Depinet, R. L. (1991). A reconsideration of testing for competence rather than for intelligence. *American Psychologist*, 1012-1024.

Barrick, M. R., & Mount, M. K. (1991). The big five personality dimensions and job performance: A meta-analysis. *Personnel Psychology, 44*, 1-26.

[Haworth co-indexing entry note]: "References." Kiraly, Meredith. Co-published simultaneously in *Child & Youth Services* (The Haworth Press, Inc.) Vol. 23, No. 1/2, 2001, pp. 125-134; and: *Residential Child Care Staff Selection: Choose with Care* (Meredith Kiraly) The Haworth Press, Inc., 2001, pp. 125-134. Single or multiple copies of this article are available for a fee from The Haworth Document Delivery Service [1-800-HAWORTH 9:00 a.m. - 5:00 p.m. (EST). E-mail address: getinfo@haworthpressinc.com].

Beedell, C., & Clough, R. (1992). *Evidence for the inquiry into the selection, development and management of staff in children's homes.* (Unpublished Manuscript)

Bernardin, H., & Pence, E. (1980). Effects of rater training: Creating new response sets and decreasing accuracy. *Journal of Applied Psychology, 65*(1), 60-66.

Bernardin, J., & Buckley, M. (1981). Strategies in rater training. *Academy of Management Review, 6*(2), 205-212.

Berridge, D. (1992a, October). *Raising the status and skills of residential and foster carers.* Paper presented at the conference, Focus on Children When Families Break Down, Wollongong NSW.

Berridge, D. (1992b, October). *The contribution of research to child welfare policy.* Paper presented at the conference Focus on Children When Families Break Down, Wollongong NSW.

Berridge, D., & Wenman, H. (1995). Involving children's centre residents in recruiting a university researcher. *Children UK*, 12-13.

Besnoff, L. (1989). Avoiding claims of negligent hiring. *Supervisory Management, August*, 11-16.

Binning, J. F., Goldstein, M. A., Garcia, M. F., Harding, J. L., & Scattaregia, J. H. (1988). Effects of preinterview impressions on questioning strategies in same- and opposite-sex employment interviews. *Journal of Applied Psychology, 73*, 30-37.

Blinkhorn, S., & Johnson, J. (1991). In C. Fletcher (Ed.), *Personality tests: The Great debate* (pp. 38-39): *Personnel Management.*

Bloom, R. B. (1992). When staff members sexually abuse children in residential care. *Child Welfare, LXXI*, 131-145.

Buckley, M. R., & Eder, R. W. (1988). B. M. Springbett and the notion of the "snap decision" in the interview. *Journal of Management, 14*(1), 59-67.

Bullock, R., Little, M., & Millham, S. (1993). *Going home: The return of children separated from their families.* UK: Dartmouth.

Burgess, D. (n.d.). *The screening of child and youth care counsellor applicants.* Unpublished manuscript.

Buzatu, G. (1987). *Report on recruitment, selection, induction practices and standards and the current turnover rates and effect of lack of permanency on youth officers and child care officers employed by Community Services-Victoria.* Melbourne.

Campion, J. E., & Arvey, R. D. (1989). Unfair discrimination in the employment interview. In R. W. Eder & G. R. Ferris (Eds.), *The Employment Interview: Theory, Research and Practice* (pp. 61-74). Newbury Park, California: Sage.

Campion, M. A., Pursell, E. D., & Brown, E. (1988). Structured interviewing: Raising the psychometric properties of the employment interview. *Personnel Psychology, 41*, 25-42.

Canadian Youth in Care Network. (1994, June 23). *The right to be heard, but is anyone listening?* Paper presented at the Family Centered Child and Youth Care Conference: International Child and Youth Care Conference, Milwaukee.

Carter, M. (1986). Securing quality staff: Will criminal history checks help? *Child Care Information Exchange*, 31-32.

Cashmore, J., Dolby, R., & McGregor, S. (1994). *Systems abuse: Problems and solutions.* Sydney: NSW Child Protection Council.

Cattel, R., Eber, H., & Tatsuoka, M. (1980). *Handbook for the sixteen personality factor questionnaire.* Champaign, Illinois: Institute for Personality and Ability Testing.

Cavanagh, J. (1991). Protocol for responding to complaints regarding the treatment of children and young people in out-of-home care. Inner Urban Region of Community Services Victoria, Melbourne: Unpublished report.

Clough, R. (1986). *Scandals in residential centres: A report to the Wagner Committee*. Bristol: University of Bristol.

Clough, R. (1994, June 22). *Quality in residential child care and education*. Paper presented at the Family Centered Child and Youth Care Conference: International Child and Youth Care Conference, Milwaukee.

Cohen, S., & Gump, H. F. (1984). Using simulations to improve selection decisions. *Training and Development Journal*, 85-88.

Colligan, R., Goke, D., & Endres, V. (1977). Objective selection of effective child care workers. *Child Care Quarterly, 6*(1), 42-50.

Commissioner for Equal Opportunity. (1978, November). Some interviewing guidelines for nondiscriminatory job selection. *Equal Opportunity Bulletin*.

Commissioner for Equal Opportunity. (1986, December). Some inappropriate questions and recommended substitute questions. *Equal Opportunity Bulletin*.

Commissioner for Equal Opportunity. (1992a). Impairment discrimination. Melbourne: Author.

Commissioner for Equal Opportunity. (1992b). *Fifteenth annual report*. Melbourne: Government Printer.

Community Services Commission. (1996). *Who cares? Protecting people in residential care*. Sydney.

Denholm, C. (1988). Hiring school-based professionals: Strategies in the selection process. *Child and Youth Care Administration* (1), 17-20.

Department of Community Welfare Services. (1985). *Review of residential child care in Victoria*. Melbourne: Author.

Department of Human Services. (1997). *The redevelopment of Victoria's youth and family services: Strategic directions*. Melbourne: Authors.

Dessler, G. (1988). *Personnel management* (4th ed.). Englewood Cliffs: Prentice-Hall.

De Witte, K. (1989). Recruiting and advertising. In P. Herriot (Ed.), *Assessment and selection in organizations–methods and practice for recruitment and appraisal* (pp. 205-217). Chichester: John Wiley and Sons.

Dill, J. (1990, December 12-14). *Child care perceiver training workshop*. Cleveland, Tennessee.

Dipboye, R. L. (1989). Threats to the incremental validity of interviewer judgments. In R. W. Eder & G. R. Ferris (Eds.), *The employment interview: Theory, research and practice* (pp. 45-60). Newbury Park, CA: Sage.

Dipboye, R., Fontenelle, G., & Garner, K. (1984). Effects of previewing the application on interview process and outcomes. *Journal of Applied Psychology, 69*(1), 118-128.

Dobson, P. (1989). Reference reports. In P. Herriot (Ed.), *Assessment and Selection in Organizations* (pp. 455-468): John Wiley and Sons.

Dreher, G. F., & Maurer, S. D. (1989). Assessing the employment interview: Deficiencies associated with the existing domain of validity coefficients. In R. W. Eder & G. R. Ferris (Eds.), *The Employment Interview: Theory, Research and Practice*. Newbury Park, CA: Sage.

ECPAT Australia. (1999). *End child prostitution, pornography and trafficking: An ECPAT resource.* Melbourne: Author.

Eder, R. W., Kacmar, K. M., & Ferris, G. R. (1989). Employment interview research: History and synthesis. In R. W. Eder & G. R. Ferris (Eds.), *The Employment Interview: Theory, Research and Practice* (pp. 17-31). Newbury Park, CA: Sage.

Equal Employment Opportunity Commission. (1978). Uniform guidelines on employee selection procedures. *Federal Register, 43*(166), 38290-38315.

Equal Employment Opportunity Coordinating Council. (1976). Federal executive agency guidelines on employee selection procedures. *Federal Register, 41*(227), 51734-51759.

Fahlberg, V. I. (1991). *A child's journey through placement.* Indianapolis, USA: Perspectives Press.

Fletcher, C. (1991, September). (ed.) Personality tests: The great debate. *Personnel Management*, 38-42.

Fletcher, C. (1992, March 5). *Performance appraisal and performance management: Myths and motivation–an inaugural lecture by Professor Clive Fletcher.* Goldsmiths' College, University of London.

Fletcher, C. (1993). Testing times for the world of psychometrics. *Personnel Management, December*, 46-50.

Fletcher, C. (1994). Validity, test use and professional responsibility. *The Psychologist*, 30-31.

Forsythe, S., Drake, M. F., & Cox, C. E. (1985). Influence of applicant's dress on interviewer's selection decisions (*sic*). *Journal of Applied Psychology, 70*(2), 374-378.

Forward, A. (1995). Breach of duty: A new paradigm of the abuse of children and adolescents in care. *Children Australia, 20*(3), 19-26.

Furnham, A., & Burbeck, E. (1989). Employment interview outcomes as a function of interviewers' experience. *Perceptual and Motor Skills, 69*, 395-402.

Gardner, D., Foo, M. H., & Hesketh, B. (1995). Realistic job previews: Information processing and the accuracy of self-assessment. *Australian Psychologist, 30*(1), 64-70.

Giffin, M. (1989). Personnel research on testing, selection and performance appraisal. *Public Personnel Management, 18*(2), 127-137.

Gilmore, D., & Ferris, G. (1989). The effects of applicant impression management tactics on interviewer judgments. *Journal of Management, 15*(4), 557-564.

Goldstein, J., Freud, A., & Solnit, A. (1973). *Beyond the best interests of the child.* New York: Free Press.

Gottfredson, L. S. (1986). Societal consequences of the g factor in employment. *Journal of Vocational Behaviour, 29*, 379-410.

Guion, R. (1989). Comments on personnel selection methods. In M. Smith & I. Robertson (Eds.), *Advances in Selection and Assessment* (pp. 112-128). Chichester UK: John Wiley and Sons.

Haddock, M. D., & McQueen, W. M. (1983). Assessing employee potentials for abuse. *Journal of Clinical Psychology, 39*(6), 1021-1029.

Hanson, T. J., & Balestreri-Spiro, J. (1985). Recruitment: An alternative to interviews. *Personnel Journal, 64*(5), 114-123.

Harris, M. M. (1989). Reconsidering the employment interview: A review of recent literature and suggestions for future research. *Personnel Psychology, 42*, 691-726.

Hart, S. N. (1989). Review of the Child Abuse Potential Inventory Form IV. *Buros Mental Measurement Year Book, No 10*, 152-153.

Health and Community Services. (1994). *Placement and support program: The vision for redevelopment*. Melbourne: Author.

Hebenton, B., & Thomas, T. (1992). The disqualification of childminders: A new form of assessment? *Children and Society*, *6*(2), 125-131.

Hebenton, B., & Thomas, T. (1994a). Under scrutiny. *Community Care*, 26-27.

Hebenton, B., & Thomas, T. (1994b). The closed world of Warner: A comment on "choosing with care." *Practice*, *7*(1), 55-62.

Hendley, B. (1994, July 12). *An integrated system for young people in residential care*. Paper presented at the Residential Child Care: Into the Next Century. Day Conference run by the National Children's Bureau of the United Kingdom (NCB-UK), London.

Herman, K. H. (1993). Enhancing screening for child and youth care work with problem-specific measures: An example with Big Brothers/Big Sisters Volunteers. *Child and Youth Care Forum*, *22*(6), 459-476.

Honig, A. (1979). What you need to know to select and train your day care staff. *Child Care Quarterly*, *8*(1), 19-35.

Hunter, J. (1986). Cognitive ability, cognitive aptitudes, job knowledge and job performance. *Journal of Vocational Behaviour*, *29*(3), 340-362.

Jamieson, S. (1994, July 1). *Social work perspectives–the way ahead*. Paper presented at the Supporting and Keeping Staff in Residential Child Care: Scotland in a European Context, Edinburgh.

Janz, T. (1982). Initial comparisons of patterned behaviour description interviews versus unstructured interviews. *Journal of Applied Psychology*, *67*(5), 577-580.

Janz, T., Hellervik, L., & Gilmore, D. (1986). *Behaviour description interviewing: New, accurate, cost effective*. Boston: Allyn and Bacon, Inc.

Jones, J. W., & Joy, D. S. (1987). *Use of the personnel selection interview for child care workers: A summary* (Technical Report No 66). Park Ridge, Illinois: London House Inc.

Jones, J. W., Joy, D. S., & Martin, S. L. (1990). A multidimensional approach for selecting child care workers. *Psychological Reports*, *67*, 543-553.

Kacmar, K. M., Ratcliff, S., & Ferris, G. R. (1989). Employment interview research: Internal and external validity. In R. W. Eder & G. R. Ferris (Eds.), *The Employment Interview: Theory, Research and Practice* (pp. 32-42). Newbury Park, CA: Sage.

Kahan, B. (1979). *Growing up in care*. United Kingdom: Blackwell.

Kahan, B. (1994, June 23). *High quality residential care?* Paper presented at the conference, Family Centered Child and Youth Care: International Child and Youth Care Conference, Milwaukee.

Kahan, B., Banner, G., & Lane, D. (1986). *Staff . . . finding them . . . choosing them . . . keeping them*. Surbiton, UK: Social Care Association.

Kahan, B., & Levy, A. (1991). *The Pindown Experience and the protection of children: Report of the Staffordshire Child Care Inquiry*: Staffordshire County Council.

Kemmis, S., & McTaggert, R. (1988). *The action research planner*. Victoria, Australia: Deakin University.

Kildonan Child and Family Services. (1999). Selecting and retaining residential child care workers. Melbourne: Author

Kiraly, M. (1994). The right to be heard, but is anyone listening? Report from the International Child and Youth Care Conference. *Children Australia, 19*(3), 33-34.

Kiraly, M. (1995). Focus groups data.

Kiraly, M. (1996). The problem of the paedophile: Guidelines for recruiting staff for positions in child and youth care. *Children Australia, 21*(2), 35-37.

Kiraly, M. (1998). *Residential child care staff selection.* Unpublished master's thesis, La Trobe University, Melbourne, Australia.

Krueger, R. A. (1988). *Focus groups: A practical guide for applied research.* Newbury Park: Sage.

Lanning, K. V. (1986). *Child molesters: A behavioral analysis.* Washington, DC: National Institute for Missing and Exploited Children.

Latham, G., Saari, L., Pursell, E., & Campion, M. (1980). The situational interview. *Journal of Applied Psychology, 65(4)*, 422-427.

Latham, G., Wexley, K., & Pursell, E. (1975). Training managers to minimize rating errors in the observation of behaviour. *Journal of Applied Psychology, 60*(5), 550-555.

Latham, J., & Saari, L. (1984). Do people do what they say? Further studies on the Situational Interview. *Journal of Applied Psychology, 59*(40), 569-573.

Lindsay, M. (1995). Involving young people in decision-making. *Children Australia, 20*(1), 39-42.

Lindsay, M., & Rayner, S. (1993). Balanced judgements. *Community Care*, 24-25.

London House Inc. (1980). Personnel Selection Inventory. Park Ridge, Illinois: Author.

London, M., & Bray, D. W. (1980). Ethical issues in testing and evaluation for personnel decisions. *American Psychologist, 35*(10), 890-901.

Loretto, V. (1986). Recruitment: Effective interviewing is based on more than intuition. *Personnel Journal, 65*(12), 101-107.

Macan, T. M., & Dipboye, R. L. (1988). The effects of interviewers' initial impressions on information gathering. *Organizational Behaviour and Human Decision Processes, 42*, 364-387.

Madge, N. (1994, July 1). *A comparative approach to residential care in Europe.* Paper presented at the conference Supporting and Keeping Staff in Residential Child Care: Scotland in a European Context, Edinburgh.

Maier, H. W. (1979). The core of care: Essential ingredients for the development of children away from home. *Child Care Quarterly, 8*(3) Fall), 161-173.

Maloney, D. M., Warfel, D. J., Blase, K. A., Timbers, G. D., Fixsen, D. L., & Phillips, E. L. (1983). A method for validating employment interviews for residential child care workers. *Residential Group Care and Treatment, 1*(4), 37-50.

Maluccio, A. N., Fein, E., & Olmstead, K. A. (1986). *Permanency planning for children: Concepts and methods.* New York: Tavistock Publications.

Maurer, S. D., & Fay, C. (1988). Effect of situational interviews, conventional structured interviews and training on interview rating agreement: An experimental analysis. *Personnel Psychology, 41*, 329-344.

McCaughan, N. (1992). Speaking out: Setting up a forum of young users. *Children and Society, 6*(3), 241-249.

McClelland, D. C. (1973). Testing for competence rather than for "intelligence." *American Psychologist, 28*, 1-14.

McLaughlin, Y., & McLean, J. (1987). *Effective staff selection (workshop handbook)*. Melbourne: David Syme Business School, Chisholm Institute of Technology.

McMenamin, B. (1996). Prevention of child sexual assault through sound employment practices: Guidelines and issues for non-government agencies. Melbourne: ECPAT Australia (End Child Prostitution, Pornography and Trafficking).

McMillan, I., Robinson, S., & King, D. (n.d.). A research-based framework for selecting residential child care workers.

Megargee, E. I. (1972). The California Psychological Inventory Handbook. San Francisco, CA: Jossey-Bass.

Melrose Film Productions. (1994). *More than a gut feeling*. London: Melrose Film Productions.

Melton, G. B. (1989). Review of the Child Abuse Potential Inventory Form IV. *Buros Mental Measurement Year Book, No 10*, 153-155.

Meyer, H. H. (1987). Predicting supervisory ratings versus promotional progress in test validation studies. *Journal of Applied Psychology, 72*(4), 696-697.

Millham, S., Bullock, R., Hosie, K., & Haak, M. (1986). *Lost in care*. United Kingdom: Gower.

Milner, J. (1986). Child Abuse Potential Inventory Manual Second Edition. DeKalb, Illinois: Psytec, Inc.

Milner, J. S., & Wimberley, R. C. (1979). An inventory for the identification of child abusers. *Journal of Clinical Psychology, 35*(1), 95-100.

Milner, J. S., & Wimberley, R. C. (1980). Prediction and explanation of child abuse. *Journal of Clinical Psychology, 36*(4), 875-884.

Moriarty, A. (1990). Deterring the molester and abuser: Pre-employment testing for child and youth care workers. *Child and Youth Care Quarterly, 19*(1), 59-66.

Muchinsky, P. (1979). The use of reference reports in personnel selection: A review and evaluation. *Journal of Occupational Psychology, 52*, 287-297.

Mufson, D. (1986). Selecting child care workers for adolescents: The California Psychological Inventory. *Child Welfare, 65*(1), 83-88.

Murphy, J. (1994). Not just a job: A study of the needs of residential child care workers in Melbourne, Australia. *Children Australia, 19*(1), 27-32.

Murray, K. (1986). Legal aspects of the selection process. *Child Care Information Exchange, January*, 27-30.

National Children's Bureau. (1994). *Induction programme for residential care*. London: Practice Development Department–Children's Residential Care Unit.

Nunno, M., & Rindfleisch, N. (1991). The abuse of children in out of home care. *Children and Society, 5*(4), 295-305.

O'Brien, T. (1994, July 1). *The COSLA Perspective–the way ahead.* Paper presented at the conference Supporting and Keeping Staff in Residential Child Care: Scotland in a European Context: Edinburgh: Children in Scotland.

Parkes, W. (1985). *Recruiting in Australia*. Frenchs Forest NSW: Reed.

Patton, M. Q. (1990). *Qualitative evaluation and research methods second edition*. Newbury Park, California: Sage.

Pearn, M., & Kandola, R. (1988). *Job analysis: A practical guide for managers*. London: Institute of Personnel Management.

Pecora, P. J., & Austin, M. J. (1987). *Managing human services personnel* (vol. 48). Newbury Park, California: Sage.

Peters, D. L., & Getz, S. F. (1986). Getting beyond the robot model of the child care worker. *Journal of Children in Contemporary Society, 17*(3), 103-111.

Peters, D., & Madle, R. (1991). The development of effective child and youth care workers. In J. Beker & A. Eisikovits (Eds.), *Knowledge Utilization in Residential Child and Youth Care Practice* (291-312). Washington, DC: Child Welfare League.

Peters, J. C., & Waterman, R. H. (1986). *In search of excellence: Lessons from America's best run companies*. Sydney: Harper and Row.

Peters, T. (1988). *Thriving on chaos: Handbook for a management revolution*. New York: Harper and Row.

Pfau, J. (1990). The ten most common interviewing mistakes. *Supervisory Management, 35*(12), 9.

Phillip Institute of Technology. (1982). *Residential child care in Victoria: Some suggestions for practice development*. Melbourne: Author.

Pringle, K. (1993). Gender politics. *Community Care, 956*, 16-17.

Pursell, E. D., Campion, M. A., & Gaylord, S. R. (1980). Structured interviewing: Avoiding selection problems. *Personnel Journal, 59*(11), 907-912.

Rasmussen, K. G. (1984). Nonverbal behaviour, verbal behaviour, resume credentials, and selection interview outcomes. *Journal of Applied Psychology, 69*(4), 551-556.

Robertson, I. R., & Makin, P. J. (1993). Selection methods and their usage. *Recruitment, Selection and Retention, 2*(1), 3-10.

Robinson, S., & King, D. (1996, 3-6 September). *A research-based framework for selecting residential child care workers*. Paper presented at the Realities and Dreams: International Conference on Residential Child Care, Glasgow.

Ross, A. L., & Hoeltke, G. (1985). A tool for selecting residential child care workers: An initial report. *Child Welfare, LXIV*(1), 46-54.

Ross, A. L., & Hoeltke, G. (1987). An interviewing tool for selection of residential child care workers: A follow-up report. *Child Welfare, LXVI*(2), 46-54.

Rowe, P. M. (1989). Unfavorable information and interview decisions. In R. W. Eder & G. R. Ferris (Eds.), *The Employment Interview: Theory, Research and Practice* (pp. 77-89). Newbury Park, California: Sage.

Saul, P. (1980). Psychological testing in the selection process. *Work and People, 6*(2), 19-22.

Saunders, B. T., & Pappanikou, A. J. (1970). Minnesota Multiphasic Personality Inventory subscale indices of effective child care personnel. *Devereux Schools Forum, 6*, 19-26.

Saville and Holdsworth Ltd. (1984). Occupational personality questionnaire (OPQ) manual. Esher, Surrey, United Kingdom: Saville and Holdsworth Limited.

Schaefer, C. (1973). Development of a new scale for selecting child care personnel. *Child Care Quarterly, 2*(2), 107-112.

Schneider, B., & Konz, A. (1989). Strategic job analysis. *Human Resource Management, 28*(1), 51-63.

Selection Research Inc. (1982). SRI Child Care Worker Perceiver. Lincoln, Nebraska.

Skinner, A. (1994, July 1). *Review of residential care in Scotland*. Paper presented at the conference Supporting and Keeping Staff in Residential Child Care: Scotland in a European Context. Edinburgh: Children in Scotland.

Smith, M. (1991). Comment in Personality Tests: The Great Debate (Ed.) Clive Fletcher, *Personnel Management* (September), 41.

South Australia Community Welfare Advisory Committee. (1973). *Enquiring into residential child care in South Australia.* Adelaide: Author.

Springbett, B. M. (1958). Factors affecting the final decision in the employment interview. *Canadian Journal of Psychology, 12,* 13-22.

Staley, C. C., Ranck, E. R., Perreault, J., & Neugebauer, R. (1986). Guidelines for effective staff selection. *Child Care Information Exchange,* 22-26.

Standing Committee of Community Services and Income Security Administrators. (1995). *National baseline standards on out-of-home care.* Canberra: Health and Community Services Ministerial Council.

Stone, R. J. (1985). Personality tests in executive selection. *Human Resource Management Australia, 23*(4), 10-14.

Support Force for Children's Residential Care. (1994). *Recruitment and selection techniques: Database.* United Kingdom.

Support Force for Children's Residential Care. (1995b). *Code of practice for the employment of residential child care workers.* United Kingdom.

Support Force for Children's Residential Care. (1995c). *Good care matters–ways of enhancing good practice in residential child care.* United Kingdom.

Tresiliotis, J., & Russell, J. (1984). *Hard to place.* United Kingdom: Heinemann.

Tucker, D. H., & Rowe, P. M. (1979). Relationship between expectancy, causal attribution and final hiring decisions in the employment interview. *Journal of Applied Psychology, 64,* 27-34.

Tullar, W. L., Mullins, L. T. W., & Caldwell, S. A. (1979). Effects of interview length and applicant quality on interview decision time. *Journal of Applied Psychology, 64*(6), 669-674.

United Kingdom Dept of Health. (1992). *Choosing with care. The Report of the Committee of Inquiry into the Selection, Development and Management of Staff in Children's Homes (Warner Report).* London: (HMSO).

United Kingdom Save the Children Fund. (1996). *Involving children and young people in recruitment.* United Kingdom: Author.

United Kingdom. (1989). *Children Act.* London, UK: HMSO.

United Nations General Assembly. (1989). *Convention on the rights of the child.*

United States of America. (1964). *Civil rights act, title VII.*

United States of America. (1972). *Equal Employment Opportunity Act.*

Utting, W. (1991). *Children in the public care: A review of residential child care.* London: HMSO.

Victorian Council of Social Service. (1993). *The community employing handbook. A guide to employment issues for community organizations.* Melbourne: Victorian Council for Social Service.

Victoria. (1989). *Children and Young Person's Act 1989.* Victorian Government Printer.

Victoria. (1995). *Equal opportunity act.*

Victorian Association of Young People in Care. (n.d.). INFO PACK. Melbourne.

Wagner, G. (1987). *Residential care–a positive choice.* London: HMSO.

Wanous, J. P. (1982). Tell it like it is at realistic job previews. In H. G. Heneman III & D. P. Schwab (Eds.), *Perspectives on Personnel/Human Resource Management* (rev. ed., pp. 133-139). Homewood, Illinois: Richard D. Irwin, Inc.

Ward, H. (Ed.) (1995). *Looking after children: Research into practice.* London: HMSO.

Wasmund, W. C., & Tate, T. T. (1988). Personality and performance: Attributes of effective residential child care workers. *Child Welfare, 67*(4), 291-299.

Wendover, R. W. (1989). *Smart hiring*. Naperville, Illinois: Sourcebooks, Inc.

Wexley, K., Sanders, R., & Yukl, G. (1973). Training interviewers to eliminate contrast effects in employment interviews. *Journal of Applied Psychology, 57*(3), 233-236.

Wiesner, W. H., & Cronshaw, S. F. (1988). A meta-analytical investigation of the impact of interview format and degree of structure on the validity of the employment interview. *Journal of Occupational Psychology, 61*, 275-290.

Willow, C. (1996). *Children's rights and participation in residential care.* London: National Children's Bureau.

Wright, P. M., Lichtenfels, P. A., & Pursell, E. D. (1989). The structured interview: Additional studies and a meta-analysis. *Journal of Occupational Psychology, 62*, 191-199.

Wyre, R. (1996, 10-11 October). *Preventing sexual abuse through organizational strategies.* Paper presented at the conference Facing the issues together: A response to sexual abuse within the Church, Melbourne.

Zedeck, S., Tziner, A., & Middlestadt, S. E. (1983). Interviewer validity and reliability: An individual analysis approach. *Personnel Psychology, 36*(2), 355-370.

APPENDICES

Appendix A

Examples of Situational and Behavioral Questions for Interviews[1]

The following questions are taken from the context of residential child care and are presented as models for situational questions for a range of work contexts.

SITUATIONAL QUESTIONS

A twelve year old boy gets on his bike in fit of rage and rides off into the night without lights on his bike. What do you do?

An asthmatic child in your care is resisting taking her medication. What would you do?

One of the young people has brought it to your attention that two of the others were involved in sexual activity the night before. What would you do? What consequences, if any, would be appropriate?

You have just given a child permission to go for a walk unsupervised. In front of the child, a co-worker disagrees with your decision and denies the permission. What would you do? What if the co-worker is your supervisor?

What would you do if a young person in the unit came up to you and said that he/she was attracted to you?

If there was a child in the house that other staff seemed to favour, how would you approach this? If there was a child that other staff seemed to pick on, what would you do?

Your co-worker has just given a child what you feel to be a stiff punishment for what you believe to be a minor matter. How would you deal with it?

If there was a child in the house that other staff seem to favour, how would you approach this? If there was a child that other staff seemed to pick on, what would you do?

Let's say the mother of a child in your care is getting really angry and looks like she is going to hit you. What would you do?

Can you think of a problem behaviour which you might select to work on with a child over a period of time. Step-by-step, what would you do?

You suspect one of the older children of stealing thirty dollars from your purse, but you can't prove it. What would you do?

A parent phones you and complains that one of your relieving staff has been calling her child a wimp. What do you say?

[Haworth co-indexing entry note]: "Appendix A." Kiraly, Meredith. Co-published simultaneously in *Child & Youth Services* (The Haworth Press, Inc.) Vol. 23, No. 1/2, 2001, pp. 135-136; and: *Residential Child Care Staff Selection: Choose with Care* (Meredith Kiraly) The Haworth Press, Inc., 2001, pp. 135-136. Single or multiple copies of this article are available for a fee from The Haworth Document Delivery Service [1-800-HAWORTH 9:00 a.m. - 5:00 p.m. (EST). E-mail address: getinfo@haworthpressinc.com].

A child is admitted to your residential unit late one afternoon, at the busy time when dinner is being prepared, children are being bathed, and the phone is ringing constantly. He crawls under a couch and refuses to come out. What would you do?

BEHAVIORAL QUESTIONS

Please tell us about a time in which a child you were responsible for did something very unexpected and worrying. What happened, and how did you handle it?

This job is a demanding one, and requires the incumbent to be very organized, and to plan carefully. Please give us an example of how you may have had to handle competing priorities by organizing the demands on you.

Can you select two children or young people with whom you have worked. Can you give one example of a successful and an unsuccessful casework relationship with the children and explain why each occurred

Have you ever worked with a kid that really got under your skin. What did you do about it?

Could you tell us about a child of whom you have been particularly fond, and why?

What are some ways you have used to motivate children? What are some ways you have fun with children?

Can you tell us about a time when you felt the least effective or were most frustrated in your efforts to deal with a conflict between yourself and a co-worker. What was the situation? What did you say and do? What made the situation difficult for you? What was the outcome of the situation? What steps have you taken to improve your skills in this area? What are the results of these efforts?

Can you tell us about the last time you took an unpopular stand among your co-workers? Who opposed it? How did you defend your position? What was the outcome of this situation? How did it affect your ongoing working relationships with those who opposed your position?

Constructive working relationships with co-workers and clients make everybody's job easier. Tell us about a relationship that started out rocky but that ended up effective.

Can you tell us about your best example of creating a feeling of special concern for a client?

Sometimes it is necessary to take reasonable risks in caring for others. Can you tell us about a time when you took a reasonable risk which brought a good result?

Can you tell us about a time when you questioned a well-established policy and produced a better outcome as a result?

It is sometimes important to be able to understand the reasons that people oppose your ideas. Can you give an example of a time when you were able to see past a hidden agenda and take effective action to overcome some resistance to an important goal?

Teamwork is extremely important in residential care. Can you please recall a time when you were strongly tempted to complain about someone behind their back, but you did something more constructive instead?

NOTE

1. This list of questions was originally written for Selecting and Retaining Residential Child Care Workers, Kildonan Child and Family Services (1999), and is reproduced with permission.

Appendix B

EEO Acceptable and Unacceptable Interview Questions[1]

Re: Legality of Employment

Unacceptable	*Acceptable*
Are you an Australian citizen?	*Do you have the legal right to live and work in Australia?*

Re: Experience

Unacceptable	*Acceptable*
Do you have any children?	*What experience do you have with children?*
How old are your children?	*Do you have other life experience which is relevant to the job?*
Do you intend to have children/more children?	*Are you over 18 and under 65?*
Are you married? *What was your maiden/married name?* *Have you ever been divorced?*	*Are you willing to undergo a Criminal Records Check if selected for the job?*
How old are you?	*Do you have any hobbies or interests which have a direct bearing on this job application?*
Have you ever been arrested?	*Are you a member of any organisation, club, society or professional group which has a direct bearing on your suitability for this job?*
What are your hobbies and interests? *What clubs to you belong to?*	
What memberships do you have?	

Re: Qualifications

Unacceptable	*Acceptable*
What year did you complete school? University?	*What is your highest educational level?*
What subjects were you most interested in at university?	*What education (if any) have you had which is directly relevant to this job?*
	(This information is better obtained on the Application Form)
	While at university, did you take any subjects which directly relate to the job you are applying for?

[Haworth co-indexing entry note]: "Appendix B." Kiraly, Meredith. Co-published simultaneously in *Child & Youth Services* (The Haworth Press, Inc.) Vol. 23, No. 1/2, 2001, pp. 137-139; and: *Residential Child Care Staff Selection: Choose with Care* (Meredith Kiraly) The Haworth Press, Inc., 2001, pp. 137-139. Single or multiple copies of this article are available for a fee from The Haworth Document Delivery Service [1-800-HAWORTH 9:00 a.m. - 5:00 p.m. (EST). E-mail address: getinfo@haworthpressinc.com].

Re: Availability to Work

Unacceptable	Acceptable
Who will look after the children while you are working?	Are there any reasons why you would not be able to attend work regularly?
Who collects the children after school?	
How will you manage to work if the children are sick or on school holidays?	
Does your religion prevent you from working weekends or holidays?	We are looking for a person who will be able to stay in the job for a minimum of two years.
Is your spouse/partner likely to be transferred?	Are there any reasons why you are unlikely to be able to stay this long?

Re: Availability at Short Notice (if required)

Unacceptable	Acceptable
Who will look after the children if you were recalled to work unexpectedly?	Would you be available to do emergency work at short notice?
How far away do you live from the residential unit?	

Re: Health

Unacceptable	Acceptable
Do you suffer from asthma/diabetes/etc.?	Do you have any physical condition or handicap which may limit your ability to perform the job you have applied for? If yes, is there something which can be done to accommodate your limitation?
Do you have any disabilities or handicaps?	
Have you had any recent or past illnesses or operations?	Are you willing to undertake a medical examination at our expense with one of our nominated doctors (male or female at your choice) if the nature of the job requires one?
What was the date of your last general medical check-up or physical examination?	

Re: Salary

Unacceptable	Acceptable
What salary do you expect?	If you are employed, are you willing to take the prevailing wage for the job you are applying for?
What is your current salary?	

Re: Simply Irrelevant

Can you give us a contact in the case of an emergency?	*This question should only be asked of the successful applicant once appointed.*
What relationship is this person to you?	
Do you own or rent your home?	
With whom do you reside? Do you live with your parents?	
Can you provide a photograph of yourself?	
Have you ever done military service?	*No acceptable substitutes for these questions.*
Where were you born?	
How tall are you?	
What does you spouse/partner think about your work?	

Questions About Childhood Questions about applicants' own childhood experiences are sometimes seen as relevant to positions in the direct care of children and young people. However, the purpose of the enquiry should not be to make a judgement about childhood experiences the applicant may have had, but to ascertain what job-related attitudes and skills they may have acquired from their experiences. Wording of questions should reflect this. Examples of appropriate questions might be:

- *Can you comment on what you have learned about looking after children from your own upbringing? What would you seek to do the same as the way you were raised? Are there things that you aim to do differently?*
- *What is important in bringing up a child?*
- *(If appropriate) What have you learned from raising your own children? How would you like to do it better if you had the time over again?*
- *What have been key life experiences that you believe will enhance your work with children and young people?*
- *Can you tell us something about what you have learned from your formal education or training in working with children and young people? Can you tell us something about what you have learned from your life experience with children and young people?*
- *Do you think it is helpful in equipping someone to work with disturbed children if they themselves have had a happy or a disrupted childhood? Can you explain why you think that way?*

NOTE

1. This list of questions was originally written for Selecting and Retaining Residential Child Care Workers, Kildonan Child and Family Services, in press, and is reproduced with permission.

Appendix C

Model Proformas for Staff Selection

C1. Job Description

NAME OF AGENCY
JOB DESCRIPTION

Job title

1. Key function

2. Context
   [Brief description of Agency and its current developments]

3. Position Objectives
   [List three or four key objectives]

4. Responsibilities
   [List in detail, including last, Undertake other duties as required]

5. Accountability
   The [job title] reports directly to the [job title of supervisor]

6. Conditions of appointment
   The position of full-time/part-time (if part-time, specify hours).
   Remuneration and conditions of appointment will be in accordance with . . .

7. Performance Criteria

[Haworth co-indexing entry note]: "Appendix C." Kiraly, Meredith. Co-published simultaneously in *Child & Youth Services* (The Haworth Press, Inc.) Vol. 23, No. 1/2, 2001, pp. 141-152; and: *Residential Child Care Staff Selection: Choose with Care* (Meredith Kiraly) The Haworth Press, Inc., 2001, pp. 141-152. Single or multiple copies of this article are available for a fee from The Haworth Document Delivery Service [1-800-HAWORTH 9:00 a.m. - 5:00 p.m. (EST). E-mail address: getinfo@haworthpressinc.com].

	ESSENTIAL	DESIRABLE
Qualifications	Membership of [professional association]	Post-graduate diploma in . . .
Job knowledge		Knowlege of . . . legislation
Skills		
Experience	At least [. . .] years experience as a professional	Experience in speciality area
Personal qualities	Examples– Warmth, communication skills, good team-work, flexibility, creativity, sense of humour, organisational skill	
Availability	Some after hours work required, usually not more than one evening per week	
Other requirements	Driver's license	
Policy expectations	Adherence to written confidentiality policy	
Pre-employment checks required	Criminal records, identity, work history, qualifications	

C2. Application Form

NAME OF AGENCY

APPLICATION FOR EMPLOYMENT

1. Position applied for

2. Name
   Preferred title

3. Address

   Telephone

4. Qualification
   [Please give your highest qualification, and any other relevant qualifications]

5. Other relevant courses completed

6. DRIVER'S LICENSE
   Do you have a current Driver's License? yes/no
   License Number:
   Probationary or Full License
   Endorsements (if any)

6. Work History

from (month & year)	to (month & year)	name of employer	type of organisation	position held

7. Special Requirements
Do you suffer from any disability, illness or injury which might affect your performance of the tasks associated with this position or necessitate us modifying the work environment (e.g., ramp, downstairs office, etc.). If yes, please give us details (Note: Equal Opportunity guidelines apply to the consideration of this information).

8. Convictions

Do you have any convictions? YES/NO

If yes, please detail below

9. Criminal Records Check

If selected for the position, are you willing to undertake a Criminal Records Check prior to an offer of employment? YES/NO

10. Special Skills and Life Experience

(Please detail any special skills or experience which you consider is relevant to your application for this position. You may go into as much detail as you wish, and attach a separate page if necessary.)

11. Referees

Please give the names of three referees who can be contacted in reference to your application. Relevant work referees are preferred, e.g., previous supervisors or line managers; if three such referees are not available, other work referees and relevant personal referees (not relatives) are acceptable. In selecting, your referees, please select as far as possible people who are able to speak objectively about your suitability for the position.

i) Name: ____________________

Occupation ____________________

Address ____________________

Phone (w) ____________________

Phone (h) ____________________

ii) Name: ____________________

Occupation ____________________

Address ____________________

Phone (w) ____________________

Phone (h) ____________________

iii) Name: ____________________

Occupation ____________________

Address ____________________

Phone (w) ____________________

Phone (h) ____________________

11. Declaration

I certify that my answer to each of the above questions is true and that the information provided is correct.

Applicant's Signature ____________________

Date ____________________

12. Please Attach a Current Curriculum Vitae

C3. Short-Listing Grid

NAME OF AGENCY

SHORT-LISTING GRID

Job title ______________ Date: ______________

Name	Qualification	Experience in specific area of job	Other relevant work experience	Unusual relevant experience (e.g., volunteer work, personal experience)	Interview yes/no/maybe

C4. Job Interview Schedule

Job ____

Date ____

1. Can you please tell us why you have applied for this position?
2. What relevant skills and experience do you have which you feel has prepared you for this position?
3. Can you please take a moment and think about a challenging situation with a . . . which you feel that you handled well. What was happening, and what did you do?
4. Now can you please tell us about another challenging situation with a . . . which, on reflection, you would have handled differently. What was happening, what did you do, and what would you differently again?
5. 5 to 9 could be a series of customised questions, including job knowledge, attitudinal, scenario, and behavioural questions.
6. ____
7. ____
8. ____
9. What is your understanding of confidentiality?
10. Although it is regrettable, there have been instances of people finding jobs in welfare in order to pursue dishonest or illegal ends. Have you ever experienced a situation like that? Have you ever worked alongside someone who was acting unprofessionally? How was it dealt with? How would you have liked to see it dealt with? What did you do? Would you do the same thing again?
11. 11-12 might be taken from the suggested questions on page 43-44 regarding child sexual abuse.
12.
13. We are currently in the process of . . . What are your thoughts about how to keep the team working together in this situation?
14. Are there any questions which you would like to ask us?

C5. Interview Performance Rating Form

NAME OF AGENCY

Rating Scales–Employment Interview

Position ______________________________

Date ______________________________

Relevant Experience	1	2	3	4	5	6	7	Don't know
Skills . . .	1	2	3	4	5	6	7	Don't know
Skills . . .	1	2	3	4	5	6	7	Don't know
Skills . . .	1	2	3	4	5	6	7	Don't know
Skills . . .	1	2	3	4	5	6	7	Don't know
Interpersonal Skills . . .	1	2	3	4	5	6	7	Don't know
Other (specify)	1	2	3	4	5	6	7	Don't know
Other (specify)	1	2	3	4	5	6	7	Don't know

Comments

____

____

____

____

____

C6. Reference Check Proforma

NAME OF AGENCY

Reference Check Proforma

Name of Applicant ________________________________

Name of Referee ________________________________

Date of Reference ________________________________

Relationship of Referee to Applicant ________________________________

Question 1. How long have you known X and in what capacity? Is he/she a personal friend?

____
____
____
____
____
____
____
____

Question 2. Can you please comment on the skills and characteristics which X may have which might be suitable for this position.

____
____
____
____
____
____
____
____

Question 3: Nobody is perfect and everyone has aspects of themselves which they need to develop or modify. Could you please comment on areas in which X may need to grow or develop?

____

____

____

____

____

Question 4. How responsive is X to supervision and direction?

____

____

____

____

____

Question 5. To your knowledge, has X ever engaged in any incident of inappropriate behaviour or abuse?

____

____

Question 6. How strongly would you recommend X for this position?

- ☐ Not at all
- ☐ With reservations
- ☐ Neither yes or no
- ☐ Recommend
- ☐ Strongly recommend
- ☐ Don't know/Can't say

Question 7. Is there anything else you would like to say with regard to X's application?

____

____

____

Question 8. Additional question (document both question and answer)

____

____

____

Reference taken by ________________________________

C7. Selection Report

NAME OF AGENCY

Selection Report

Date of report ______________________________

Recruitment commenced ______________________________

Recruitment completed ______________________________

Job title ______________________________

Names and professional positions of people on the selection panel

____

____

Selection methods used and dates

____

____

Comments on selection process

____

____

Any changes recommended for future recruitments

____

____

Name of successful applicant ______________________________

Attachments	The job description and key selection criteria Interview proforma Reference Check proforma Proforma for any other selection method used
Confidential section (to be destroyed after a year)	The completed short-listing grid Names of short-listed applicants Rating forms completed on each short-listed applicant The applications of the short-listed applicants

Appendix D

Profile of a Skilled Residential Child Care Worker

A PERSONALITY TYPE OR A CLUSTER OF SKILLS?

According to Professor Jerry Beker (personal communication, 1994) the hardest part of the process of identifying skilled residential child care staff is knowing what to look for. Earl Stuck (personal communication, 1994) who was in 1994 Director of Residential Care Services with the Child Welfare League of America, also claims that most administrators in residential care do not know what skills residential workers need to have. He suggests that they tend to focus on personality rather than skills and see little difference between a good residential child care worker and a "nice person." Beedell and Clough (1992) take this view a step further:

> Equally important is the fact that it is difficult to answer the question "What makes a good residential worker?". . . In default of a theory people tend to fall back on a package of simplistic analogies: the warm, caring substitute Mother, the Nanny. . .This contributes to a notion that anyone can do such work. . . .

It is probably not possible to separate out completely the distinction between personality and skill profile. However, it is important to identify the profile of skills and attributes which make for a skilled residential child care worker.

THE ROLE OF INTELLIGENCE AND THE ABILITY TO LEARN

The lack of recognition of the intellectual cluster of skills required to do the job leaves us in the victim field. VanderVen (personal communication, 1994) claims that this is a cognitive, not an affective field, and that there is a whole cognitive cluster of skills required for effective residential child care work. This emphasis on the role of intelligence in effective residential child care is consistent with a large body of research on personnel selection which concludes that general cognitive ability has high validity in predicting both performance and training success in all jobs. The data collected on this topic also pointed to the importance of conceptual skills in the profile of a skilled residential child care worker. This new emphasis on the role of intelligence and the ability to learn is consistent with the increasing concern in the residential child care field across the world to see residential child care workers adequately trained, and the keenness of many to see it professionalised.

USES OF A PROFILE OF A SKILLED RESIDENTIAL CHILD CARE WORKER

This profile may be useful for developing:

> The person specification for recruitment of residential care workers.
>
> Key performance indicators for staff selection.

[Haworth co-indexing entry note]: "Appendix D." Kiraly, Meredith. Co-published simultaneously in *Child & Youth Services* (The Haworth Press, Inc.) Vol. 23, No. 1/2, 2001, pp. 153-157; and: *Residential Child Care Staff Selection: Choose with Care* (Meredith Kiraly) The Haworth Press, Inc., 2001, pp. 153-157. Single or multiple copies of this article are available for a fee from The Haworth Document Delivery Service [1-800-HAWORTH 9:00 a.m. - 5:00 p.m. (EST). E-mail address: getinfo@haworthpressinc.com].

Standard *proformas* for rating performance on selection assessments such as interviews, work tests and reference checks.

Interview and reference check questions, and work tests and exercises.

Performance appraisal tools.

Development of the profile of a skilled residential child care worker.

FINDINGS FROM THE FOCUS GROUPS

Several focus group questions directed attention towards the characteristics of a skilled child care worker. Participants in the focus groups noted that this was not an easy issue and that many people with many different personalities will be good at the job. Moreover, they expressed the view that a diversity of personalities is important to give children and young people some choice about who they wish to relate to. The comment was also made by a residential worker that the process of identifying a skilled worker will not always be one that can be clearly articulated. This has implications for selection processes, which cannot be made to be too "neat" or "scientific." In fact, a crystal ball was suggested as the best way to identify skilled staff!

Nevertheless, when the various responses were analyzed, they yielded a clear picture of the constellation of factors which participants felt were needed for the task. To analyze this data, all the various responses describing qualities or skills seen as essential or desirable were listed. Themes were sought among this data and categories established for all the responses. These categories were refined during the process. Eventually, all the descriptive labels were grouped under twelve themes. Particular descriptive phrases were selected that summarized the responses collected under each theme. These twelve themes are described below.

FINDINGS FROM THE STUDY TOUR

Expert informants were asked what they saw as the qualities necessary and/or desirable in a skilled residential child care worker. (One couple experienced in foster care described their views about the qualities needed in foster care. Most of these echoed others' views about residential care; where they varied, the additional ideas were not included). This material was added to the data collected from the focus groups and further descriptive phrases were added as appropriate. Categories were modified as necessary to reflect the additional data.

FINDINGS FROM THE LITERATURE

Many references were found which detailed the qualities needed in residential child care work. Some of these were studies utilizing psychological tests or other structured assessment methods; other articles documented opinions based upon practice wisdom. In addition, Barrick and Mount (1991) identified several personality factors that appear to be related to job performance in a general way. These were also added to data set gathered from the focus groups and the study tour.

FINDINGS FROM THE PILOT PROJECT

The pilot project (see Chapter 7) consisted of a series of staff selection exercises that involved young people or parents. Trial 1 was a process of involving young people ex-care in the recruitment of relief residential child care workers.

During the briefing and preparation session prior to the interviews, the young people were asked their views on what qualities they would look for in staff. These views have also been incorporated into the profile outlined below.

CHARACTERISTICS OF A SKILLED RESIDENTIAL CHILD CARE WORKER

The twelve characteristics of a skilled residential child care worker break down into a set of essential and a set of desirable characteristics. All can be improved by experience and training. A skilled residential child care worker is likely to display all of the necessary characteristics and some of the desirable ones.

A. Essential

Appropriate motivation and commitment

A real sense of commitment
A view that "it's more than just a job"
Clear, transparent motives
A sense of mission
Genuine interest in children and young people
"Stickability"; willingness to hang in through difficult times with children
A wish to provide continuity of interest in children beyond the length of employment

Caring

Nurturing
Empathic
A friend to children and young people, liking of them in general
An ability to make them feel safe and secure
Persistent caring (but not self-sacrifice)
Encouraging
Supportive

Flexible

Tolerant
Understanding
Accepting; treats children as individuals
Non-judgmental
Respectful
Patient
Able to give children space and choices
Able to question oneself and learn from others
Not too much programming

Resilient

A positive outlook and self-concept; optimistic; pro-social
Lots of stamina, endurance, "stickability"
Assertive
Secure
Able to handle pressure
Able to set limits and boundaries

To have a support network outside of work
Patience and self-control
Able to know one's own limits and ask for help or respite
Able to withstand being disliked by children and young people at times
Experience of personal difficulties is an advantage if resolved
Willing to be emotionally involved but also able to step back

Genuine

Honest
Open
Trustworthy
Fair and consistent
Likes children and young people, is interested in them
Clear motivation and commitment

Conceptual thinker

A knowledge base to draw on; understanding of child development; a frame of reference to work from
Reflective
Able to question one's work and learn from others
Insightful
Good problem-solving skills
A lateral thinker
Creative, curious, willing to learn
Common sense
Ability to translate knowledge into a consistent pattern of behaviour

Good communication skills

A good listener
Good problem-solving skills
Involving children and young people in decision-making about their lives
Assertiveness
Ability to communicate concerns directly and comfortably to children, and also to parents and colleagues
Understanding children's underlying needs
Taking children seriously

B. Desirable

Fun

A sense of humor
Enjoyment of one's work

Team player

Cooperative
Supportive of other staff
Good problem-solving skills

Organized

Able to maintain a good environment
Able to deal with multiple demands
Able to prioritize
Domestically competent

Experienced in relevant areas

Experience of working with children and young people
Life experience, especially with children and young people
Experience of personal problems of benefit, if resolved

The intangible and non-traditional

A person may lack some of the skills listed above but have other special qualities which are harder to define, but make for good care. A wide range of backgrounds and disciplines may lead to creative ways to relate effectively to children and young people.

Index

For Product Safety Concerns and Information please contact our EU representative GPSR@taylorandfrancis.com
Taylor & Francis Verlag GmbH, Kaufingerstraße 24, 80331 München, Germany

www.ingramcontent.com/pod-product-compliance
Lightning Source LLC
LaVergne TN
LVHW021109300926
849160LV00009B/661

* 9 7 8 0 7 8 9 0 1 7 4 5 1 *